# STUTTERING
## Therapy for Children

Prentice-Hall International, Inc., *London*
Prentice-Hall of Australia, Pty., Ltd., *Sydney*
Prentice-Hall of Canada, Ltd., *Toronto*
Prentice-Hall France, S.A.R.L., *Paris*
Prentice-Hall of India (Private) Ltd., *New Delhi*
Prentice-Hall of Japan, Inc., *Tokyo*
Prentice-Hall de Mexico, S.A., *Mexico City*

*Harold L. Luper*

Head, Department of Audiology and Speech Pathology
University of Tennessee

*Robert L. Mulder*

Director, Speech and Hearing Center
Oregon College of Education

# STUTTERING

## Therapy for Children

Prentice-Hall, Inc. *Englewood Cliffs, New Jersey*

Current printing (last digit):

12   11   10   9   8   7   6

Library of Congress Catalog Card No.: 64-13250

Printed in the United States of America (C-85898)

To our respective wives to whom we now return if they will have us back, and to our children who we fondly hope still remember us.

# Preface

This book has been written because the authors frequently receive requests for information from public school speech therapists who are discouraged about their ability to help children who stutter. These requests for information take various forms, but they invariably point up strong pressures besetting the therapist who attempts to provide for the welfare of the stuttering child: *We need to help because we are expected to help. We hesitate to help because we may cause the stuttering to worsen. We are undecided about the form our help should take because we don't know which "horse to back" when it comes to choosing among the several available theories accounting for stuttering behavior.*

Whether only one horse is backed or several, most theories of stuttering help in our understanding of *why* a child's life gets snarled up, but they say little to the student about *how* to go about the unraveling process. The prominent expositions in our literature which do provide information about therapy dwell mostly on those developmental stages of stuttering which are not commonly found in our public schools, namely the child who is just beginning to stutter, or the most advanced stages of chronic stuttering. Usually these children are either preschoolers or have graduated from high school. Although this text also includes methods and procedures suitable for the management of these "out-of-school" segments of the stuttering population, therapy for school-age children who stutter is given equal attention.

The important search for a better understanding of the *why* of stuttering continues and must continue because all of the answers are not in. This book, however, emphasizes the equally important *how*—how to help the child who stutters to modify his behavior so as to make the most of his potential without being burdened by stuttering. This book is designed as a practical book for practitioners of therapy, and the authors offer an operational approach to the management of stuttering.

This operational approach to therapy is justified on the basis of

vii

its successful application in actual speech therapy sessions in college and public school settings. The authors feel that the basic ingredients for the successful modification of stuttering are contained herein, but the exact proportions and the time and the place for appropriate action must be supplied by the reader. What is offered represents successful therapy approaches distilled from a number of tested approaches both successful and unsuccessful.

We are aware that further research and new discoveries may pave the way to better means of helping children who stutter to better speech. The authors assume that the readers have a basic understanding of the theories of stuttering causation. The reader should realize that although our purpose is to provide for the welfare of the stuttering child, we realize that all of what is written here is vulnerable to expanded, improved knowledge of this complex phenomenon.

We are especially indebted to several people who have in every sense of the word made possible the preparation of this book. Dr. Stanley Ainsworth and Dr. Walter Snyder through their understanding support and the warmth of their friendship have made this venture into print possible. The authors wish also to express their appreciation to their students and fellow staff members, at the University of Georgia and at the Oregon College of Education, who offered critical suggestions and encouragement during the formative stages of this book. To Dr. Charles Van Riper we ascribe both our basic interest in stuttering therapy and the groundwork for any important insights we may have acquired along the way. Appreciation is expressed to Mr. Malcolm Fraser and the *Speech Foundation of America* for providing opportunities and experiences conducive to professional growth and increased understanding of the problem of stuttering and to Mrs. Ruth Stump who provided the strong measure of discipline and determination necessary to keep our efforts goal-directed. We especially acknowledge the untiring efforts of Mrs. Hollis Barnes and Mrs. Ruth Hilterbrand who helped us in the preparation of the manuscript for publication.

This book is a true admixture of ideas and efforts. Because of this there is no senior author.

Acknowledgement is also made to the several publishers who have granted us permission to include quotations from their publications.

H. L. L.
R. L. M.

# Table of Contents

           (Phase One)                                          36

           Environmental Therapy for Incipient Stut-
           tering  38

           The Therapist as a Source of Information
           39

           *Disfluency as a normal part of learning to talk—39.
           The development of stuttering—41. Misconceptions
           about stuttering—42. The why of stuttering—43.
           Speech and language development—43. Bibliotherapy
           —46.*

           The Reception of the Information    47

           *Parental concern—47. Authority—50. Providing in-
           formation about stuttering—51.*

           Provision for a Course of Indirect Action
           52

           *Providing advice about problems of child care which
           are not directly speech centered—58. Counseling pro-
           cedures—60.*

           Direct Versus Environmental Therapy Ap-
           proaches  62

           Factors in Making Decisions as to the Rela-
           tive Degree of Directive Therapy Ap-
           proaches to Use  65


*Four*      The Modification of Transitional Stuttering
           (Phase Two)                                          68

           Planning for Systematic Therapy   69

           Parent Counseling  71

           *Fluency versus disfluency—73. Disfluency—74. Flu-
           ency—75.*

           Therapy Specifics  75

           Providing a Program of General Speech Im-
           provement  78

           *Desensitization therapy—83.*

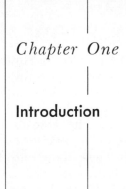

*Chapter One*

Introduction

*An operational approach to therapy for children who
stutter is described. Some of the necessary basic ingredients for the eventual modification of stuttering are
noted.*

## An Operational Approach to Therapy

*Our Interest in Stuttering*

The problem of stuttering has unflaggingly held the interest of speech pathologists since the beginning days of the profession. Why should so much attention focus on this particular type of disordered speech?

One of the most obvious reasons is that stuttering intrigues because of its complexity. Those who stutter do so in a variety of ways. Some show only fleeting signs of distress; others flounder helplessly, entangled in a web spun of their own words. Adults stutter differently from children, and, although stuttering begins most often in childhood, the adult form rarely resembles its precursor. The stutterer's life goals and his stuttering are shaped one by the other. Some forms of stuttering arouse scepticism in those who observe it because of the seemingly impractical, fantastic ways the stutterer tries to achieve ordinary, common ends. Both the stutterer and his observer are inevitably enthralled by the dramatic changes in the stutterer's behavior. Note this college student's reaction to stuttering.

> The first stutterer I ever remember seeing was the one who came in to talk to our class last time. I didn't believe it when he said he was a severe stutterer. The way he gave his report didn't stack up with what he kept saying he was really like. He looked normal and talked just the way I talk when I have to give a report, but he said he could hardly talk when he started his speech therapy. After class I stopped him in the hall; I couldn't remember his name, so I asked him. Up to that time he had been smiling and talking quite easily to someone else, when suddenly his eyes sort of rolled up and he made a sound like "uh" over and over. It went up higher in pitch every time he said it. It must have gone up more than an octave before he got his name out. Perspiration was standing way out on his forehead and I felt like I had pulled a real blunder.

The radical change in behavior between a child's active stuttering and his fluency is often so dramatic that it captures our attention. Couple this with the apparent depth of the stutterer's concern and the degree to which his life is affected and we probably have the reason why we become so involved in the stutterer's "problem." We sympathize with the stutterer's forcing and struggling, which seem so unnecessary and painful. Because he so often shows signs of being able to talk well, we feel that he can be helped and so we find ourselves trying to help. Most of us have experienced stage fright at one time or another. We cannot help feeling that stuttering is an exaggerated form of the same thing and thus we sense a kinship in anxiety. We feel strongly that there but for the grace of God talk I.

Although sympathy and understanding are worthy motivations for good speech therapy, well-intentioned efforts to help can sometimes make stuttering worse when sympathy and understanding are all that is proffered. The purpose of this book is to provide speech therapists with better weapons and less naïveté in their attempts to help a child out of his conflict.

## Operational Therapy

The contents of this book recommend a course of action that will result in a change for the better in the stutterer's behavior. The type of action recommended will vary from child to child and from age group to age group depending on awareness, concomitant emotionality, intelligence, and countless other factors. In some instances action may necessarily take the form of environmental manipulations such as counseling parents, removing disturbing influences, or modifying the expectations of listeners. Action may require actually confronting the stutterer with feared words, tremors, audience penalties, and the like. Action may be an attempt to eliminate inappropriate phonetic attacks on words and replace them with suitable alternates. Action may refer to conscious attempts to bring about attitudinal changes and improved self-understanding. In other words, the contents of this book provide a practical course of action for the practitioner.

### The Nature of Responsible Therapy

A speech therapist adventures into new territory every time he begins therapy with a child who stutters. There are many "unknowns." Every child presents a special problem of his own. With experience the therapist recognizes similarities in the difficulties encountered by children and he learns that he can make some

safe generalizations about them. But experience also teaches the
therapist to be prudent and to qualify his inferences and deductions
so as to leave an "out" in his thinking and actions when new
evidence is presented. Note how our thinking about a problem
must shift as new evidence is presented:

*Evidence.* Male—16 years of age—stutters severely. Says that so far
as he knows, he had never stuttered until he was 11 years of age.
Says that he was horseback riding alone on his parents' ranch in
New Mexico in defiance of strict orders that he was never to venture
out of sight of his ranch house alone. When he was far out of
sight of the ranch house, his horse stumbled and he was thrown to
the ground. The horse raced off and returned to the ranch house.
He pulled himself up on an outcropping of rock so that if anyone
noticed his horse returning they would be better able to see him
when they came out looking for him. His ankle had been broken
in the fall, and by the time he had pulled himself up to a place
where he could sit down, his ankle was painfully swollen and he
discovered he was sitting over a den of rattlesnakes. In great pain,
he sat in the glaring sun for more than five hours, not daring to
move for fear of falling into the writhing snakes below. He claims
he was delirious when his rescuers found him and that he stuttered
badly from that time until he began his speech therapy.

*Generalization:* This terrifying experience would be enough to
traumatize anyone into stuttering. Couple this with his guilt about
disobeying the injunction that he not ride out away from the
ranch house alone and you have a clear-cut case of stuttering precipitated by shock.

*Additional Evidence:* Case history data indicated that the boy's last
name differed from that of his mother. Questioning indicated that
his mother and father were divorced at the time of the snake pit
episode and the mother had since remarried. Conditions of the
divorce settlement provided that the boy was to spend his summer
vacation months with his father. During the remainder of the year
he was to stay with his mother who lived in a northern midwest
state. He did not return to his father's ranch the next summer.

*Revised Generalization:* Perhaps stuttering had been precipitated
during the summer he spent on his father's ranch, but the climate
for speech breakdown may have been present due to previous difficulty adjusting to his parents' separation.

*Additional Evidence:* A check of his school records disclosed the
following inconclusive but interesting information.

First grade report: ". . . nervous . . . talks very rapidly . . . referred for speech help. Speech therapist felt there was no problem."

Second grade report: "Words jumbled up, but does not stutter."

Third grade report: "Moody. Talks a great deal some days—then may be very quiet. Seems to think faster than he can talk and words pile up. Speech therapist has observed him twice during the year but does not think he should be placed in speech class."

*Revised Generalization:* Innuendo in school records may point to the availability of hesitant if not outright stuttered speech prior to claimed onset date.

*Additional Evidence:* Mother refers to summer experience in New Mexico:

"I just knew something like that would happen. I didn't want him to go that summer, and I made sure that he didn't have to go again. What I could tell you about that boy's father!"

Mother in answer to question about the possibility that he stuttered before that eventful summer:

"He always did think faster than he could talk. But it wasn't stuttering. Not till he came home from New Mexico. . . . Sometimes I'd tell him (before that summer) to think of what he wanted to say and then he would talk perfectly fine. . . . When I finally got him home he could hardly say a word!" Mother referring to the boy's father: "We never talk about that man!"

Responsible therapy is demanding. It demands that the therapist make safe generalizations about the children under his guidance so that these generalizations may be incorporated into therapy. Stated quickly, responsible therapy requires a beginning plan, or over-all goal, which will permit the successful accomplishment of subgoals. In order to make successful plans, the therapist must have special information and insights about the nature of stuttering and special methods and procedures for treating it. But if therapy is to be successful, it must be evaluated continually. Whether or not therapy is going according to plan, a careful evaluation will result in revisions which lead back to a reconsideration of the over-all plan, subgoals, methods, etc. Thus, responsible therapy is not static; it is constantly changing.

Responsible therapy is not achieved through one plan, one goal, one method, one approach, but by several of each. Therapy plans must be arrived at thoughtfully and deliberately. The plans must be carried out reasonably and flexibly and the evaluation must be conducted honestly and humanely. The burden of responsibility for the conduct of therapy must be carried by the therapist, but if the therapy is at all successful the credit must go to the child, his parents, and teachers—but only if it is successful.

The therapist must know when therapy is successful and when

it has become unproductive. He must be wise enough to terminate therapy when the child is capable of making his own unsupported adjustment or when conditions no longer favor positive results.

The details of therapy will be spelled out throughout the remaining pages of this book and are only hastily mentioned here. It must be pointed out here, however, that the remission of stuttering symptoms is only one of several criteria for successful therapy. Whenever this goal is attainable, every reasonable effort should be made to achieve it. But this goal is not attainable through the therapist's ingenuity, insight, and resolve alone. Only a few of the reward and penalty systems that induce and perpetuate stuttering behavior can be manipulated through therapy procedures. The therapist must be aware of the existence of strong demands for fluency in our society, and he must be able to help a child withstand these intense pressures while helping to repair or strengthen his impaired confidence in speaking.

## Ideal Therapy Conditions

Although responsible therapy is always demanding, it is rarely if ever conducted under ideal conditions. What are ideal therapy conditions—if there are such things? Ideal therapy conditions would allow sufficient time for therapy to be conducted in a setting and atmosphere conducive to therapy. Ideally the child would be scheduled at the request of the therapist instead of the way it usually turns out: the child scheduled on the basis of what he can best afford to miss while absent from his classroom, or squeezed into a heavy case load crowded with children who have articulation and voice problems also in urgent need of attention. The setting for therapy would permit privacy for parent conferences and for individual and group therapy sessions and would permit spatial and temporal access to the child's parents and teachers and to the child's real life, both home and school, so that therapy would not be restricted to therapist-child contacts.

This is the ideal—remote, elusive, and rarely completely attainable. One condition was left out deliberately. In an ideal therapy setting everyone involved—child, parents, teachers, school administrators—would cooperate enthusiastically. But, if everyone involved were enthusiastic, conscientious, cooperative, and highly motivated, schedules, therapy settings, time factors, etc., would be relatively unimportant because many of the conditions setting off or maintaining the stuttering might be magically dissolved and, presto, stuttering therapy would be relatively easy—which it certainly is not. Cooperation in a therapy program is much sought after because it often spells the difference between success and failure. In a condition of "complete cooperation" the principals involved would be actively engaged in trying to permit their perceptions and convictions to be changed. But cooperation is seldom equally active for all the necessary participants. Cooperation is rarely automatic. The therapist's task is to bring about changes in attitudes, conceptions, or evaluations. Stuttering therapy is an educative process. The therapist must work diligently to create a condition (often in the face of appalling odds) wherein learning can take place. But, effective therapy often occurs under substantially less than ideal conditions. The effectiveness of the therapy is often directly related to the ingenuity and resourcefulness of a therapist who recognizes the important role he must play in the education of a number of people. *But,* inevitably, the therapist finds that he cannot always be effective in therapy. Conditions are rarely ideal, and the therapist must know when conditions are such that the possibility of effective therapy is extremely remote.

## Nonideal Therapy Conditions*

Sometimes when a child who stutters is referred for therapy, the chances for working effectively with him are extremely limited. Therapy may not be too successful for one or more of the following reasons.

1. *Time.* The therapist may have a case load too heavy to permit enough time for more than a few minutes per week. The child may have regular dental appointments that take him away from his class work.
2. *Severity or complexity of speech symptoms.* Therapy may be unsuccessful because the symptoms are too severe or complex or because they are not severe or complex enough to motivate change.
3. *Degree of emotional involvement.* The child may not be aware of his problem in which case there is a danger that therapy will precipitate awareness. Or the child may be so acutely aware of his difference that he refuses to allow the therapist to work with him.
4. *Lack of cooperation by parents, teachers, or others involved.*
5. *Competing environmental conditions.* Therapy may interfere with

---

* The conditions listed in this section were adapted from a lecture by Dr. Frank Robinson presented at a meeting of the *Oregon Speech and Hearing Association,* May 1961, and are included with his permission.

extracurricular activities such as football practice or a job on a school
paper.

6. *Presence of too many competing problems, any one of which actually
   may be more important than stuttering at this time.* The child may
   have an articulation problem, a reading problem, or others.

7. *Therapy limited to actual contact with child.* Lack of cooperation or
   scheduling difficulties may make it impossible to arrange conferences
   with parents or teachers.

8. *Difficulties arranging for group sessions.* These may be due to scheduling or transportation problems.

9. *Insufficient intelligence to grasp principles of therapy or to acquire
   necessary insights.*

10. *Nature of problem indicates need for long term or depth psycho-
    therapy which most speech therapists are unable to provide.*

All of these can be resolved sufficiently to make successful therapy possible with a satisfactory portion of the children involved.
Problem number nine can be resolved in many instances by a
modification of therapy procedures, and number ten can be resolved by making appropriate referrals.

The speech therapist must decide whether to tackle the child's
problem. He may find that he does not want to because of some
of the reasons listed above, because of his belief in a prevalent
professional philosophy that direct measures will remove only the
outward symptoms of an inner conflict, because of a felt lack of
adequate preparation for work with stutterers, or because it is too
difficult to arrange for the necessary time.

When the decision is "no" there are some alternate solutions
that can be considered. Some states have provided centers where
appropriate treatment is provided by selected speech therapists.
Special summer clinics are organized to meet these particular
needs. Some communities have established centers where children
or parents are taken by the school speech therapist for examination
or interviews; therapy is cooperatively planned so that it may be
conducted by the referring therapist in his own working area.
Some school systems have successfully designated certain members
of the speech therapy staff to serve as "stuttering specialists" and
have made appropriate adjustments in case load and release time.

Sometimes "direct" treatment is postponed. Treatment is conducted on an indirect basis until conditions are more appropriate
for direct therapy.

Robinson points out, "No system of speech therapy for the

younger stutterer in a public school setting is likely to work without an intensive, general educational program for teachers, principals, superintendents, physicians, PTA groups, school nurses, and anyone else likely to be critical of 'that speech therapist who isn't doing anything about that poor little Thompson boy—the one who stutters so badly!' "

### Therapy as Concentrated Effort

In our society there is a belief that anything worthwhile can be accomplished with concentrated effort—the impossible requires only a little more time. This faith in concentrated effort is learned at an early age, and it may work to the advantage or disadvantage of progress in stuttering therapy. Some parents who subscribe to this view stubbornly stick with it and make totally unreasonable demands of their children, and their children burn themselves out trying to fulfill their parents' desires. Children who are caught in the grips of this view struggle and splutter even after they are adults, striving manfully and valiantly to "overcome" their stuttering, unfortunately unaware that there are many ways of achieving the "impossible" and that concentrated effort can take many forms.

Therapy is a form of concentrated effort, but its effort is intellectual as well as emotional and is expressed in understanding and experimentation, restraint and testing, confirmation and re-evaluation. Concentrated effort in therapy requires flexibility, and the ability of both the child and the therapist to use failure as a tool for shaping success. The therapist must be able to teach the child whom he guides that failure is the key to greater understanding of himself and of what he can accomplish. Failure helps the therapist to select the next or better approach or method. The child is taught to use failure to help him recognize the futility of continuously using a particular maladaptive behavior whether it be attitude or mannerism. He is taught to use failure as a good reason for trying something else. The therapist realizes that there are many unknowns in the therapy process, but he attempts to work on an experimental basis: observe—judge—alter—and then try again. He perseveres, but in several different ways. Coping with unknowns under conditions in which it is necessary to "take a chance" does not mean that the work is undertaken without a plan or without knowing what one is doing. We cope with "unknowns" in most areas of life. Paul Tillich (1) describes a willingness "to take a chance" in religion as an essential element of faith. Parents, whether they like it or not, operate on the basis of chance in attempting to raise their children. There are few hard and fast, safe rules to follow in child training—or anywhere in life. What most of us do to keep going is summon up our best judgment of what to do and act on that basis. We are often wrong. Most of us never know when we are wrong; those of us who are lucky enough to know we have failed, and are also blessed with the ability to take a chance and try something else in response to failure, are blessed indeed.

The therapist must know, however, that above all, therapy means responsibility, and his main responsibility is knowing what he and the child under his care are doing, and why.

*Suggestion in Therapy*

Suggestion is always an active component of therapy. Once a therapist agrees to take on the responsibility of therapy he has made an unspoken admission to the child and his parents that something positive will happen. The best wishes of all usually go with the therapist and the child as they start into therapy. This aura of wishful thinking that therapy will accomplish something often has a positive but transitory effect on the child. Some children even stop stuttering after only a few therapy sessions. Most children and their parents are lifted in spirit and feel encouraged because something good is going to happen.

But stuttering behavior is notoriously susceptible to fluctuations and remissions and markedly dependent on altered circumstances. The therapist must realize that any suggestion of a change for the better will often result in improvement—at least temporarily. Children in the early stages of stuttering are more susceptible to suggestion than are those who have stuttered longer and more anxiously. But all succumb to it in some degree. This works to an advantage in therapy in the early stages of stuttering, especially if the child's parents come to feel that "it wasn't serious after all." However, whenever the root pressures, the conflicts, the unreasonable responses to unreasonable demands either internal (induced by the child) or external (induced by the child's parents, teachers, or others) remain unchanged, the benefits accruing from the suggestive effects of therapy will soon wear off either during the course of therapy or at the termination of therapy.

Suggestion as a method of therapy should be used judiciously. In Chapter Four, suggestion is recommended as an appropriate approach to the modification of stuttering symptoms when they are at a certain level of development. The therapist should know that suggestion will be encountered in therapy and that he cannot always be certain when it is operating. Its presence sometimes makes many of the threatening and more emotionally demanding therapy approaches and methods more palatable to a child. But it should be recognized for what it is. The fluency that comes after the introduction of a new method may be the result of the new method's suggestive value to the child. Too often, we find that some methods aren't really "working" at all, but suggestion is.

The authors are aware that almost any novel approach used decisively and with a display of confidence in its infallibility will garner some change in stuttering behavior. The procedures outlined in the following chapters will work through suggestion if for no other reason. These procedures, however, are not set forward as an easy way to a quick cure—we offer no magic—they are painstaking efforts to provide a real measure of increased self-confidence in the ability to talk for children who stutter.

## Stuttering Therapy Is Rewarding

Some of the greatest satisfactions in the practice of speech therapy come from efforts to help children who stutter. It is rewarding to be able to help instill courage and to help head off fear. As the child's overt abnormalities decrease and disappear and as he experiences the true joy of talking spontaneously without restraint, we reap the rewards of responsible therapy.

### The Contents of Later Chapters

Following is a brief summary of the contents of the chapters of this book.

## Provision for a Differential Diagnosis

Because stuttering goes through developmental changes from its inception to its most advanced stages, the noticeable features involved in these changes are discussed so as to permit adequate diagnosis and evaluation. At least four developmental stages are noted and discussed in terms of the characteristic symptoms and features. Chapter Two is devoted to a discussion of the diagnosis and evaluation of stuttering. Each of the chapters concerned with therapy procedures reviews the salient features of stuttering at the particular level or development under discussion.

*Provision for Differential Therapy*

Therapy procedures vary for each developmental stage. In the earliest developmental stages of stuttering, the child is not usually directly involved in a therapist-child relationship. At some stages of development, the child has not developed deep-seated fears of words and speaking situations and, consequently, therapy procedures differ from those stages where the child is desperately embarrassed by his verbal frustrations. These therapy procedures do not emphasize a single method. Several serviceable methods are advocated to be employed in concert to serve the needs of the child who stutters, whatever his level of difficulty.

*Provision for a Rationale*

Because an understanding of the nature of stuttering is necessary in order to plan for remedial work, part of each chapter concerned with therapy is devoted to a discussion of the significant aspects of stuttering characteristics of a particular level. Also, an attempt is made to provide for an accounting of the rationale for each therapy procedure so as to provide better understanding of the advantages and disadvantages of each approach to therapy.

*Reference*

1. TILLICH, P., *Dynamics of Faith* (New York: Harper & Row, Publishers, 1958).

*Chapter Two*

## Diagnosis and Evaluation of
## the Child Who Stutters

*This chapter is concerned with the ways of detecting and systematically reporting overt and covert manifestations of stuttering. A properly oriented diagnostic and evaluative program is not only considered to be the basis for successful modification of stuttering, but is viewed as the actual starting place for stuttering therapy.*

In order to plan for therapy it is reasonable to obtain answers to questions such as the following:

1. Is the person's speech properly identified as stuttering?
2. Should measures be initiated to modify the person's speech or behavior?
3. If so, should these measures be primarily environmental manipulations or should they involve doing something directly with the speaker?
4. If environmental therapy is planned, which person or persons can best help with the changes? What types of changes are needed and what types are possible?
5. If therapy is to involve direct contact between the therapist and the child, should the therapy be such that the child would be made more aware of the problems of stuttering or should the child be kept unaware of any emphasis upon speech and stuttering?
6. If speech patterns need modification, which aspects should receive consideration?
7. If the individual's fears of speech situations need to be decreased, which fears need the greatest attention?

## When Is Stuttering Stuttering?

It is difficult to give a definite answer to this question. When a child's parents or his teacher say the child is stuttering he may actually be stuttering or it may be that stuttering-like behaviors mark his speech. Sometimes the significant difference, at the onset of stuttering, may be in the number of the stuttering-like occurrences, or sometimes, as Johnson (14) has indicated, the difference may lie in the ear of the observer; that is, it may be that the observer is unnecessarily concerned about the same types of disfluencies as found in the speech of many young children, but which are not the forerunners of stuttering. The real problem in diagnosis at the apparent onset of stuttering is to determine whether conditions (either in the child, or his environment, or both) are ripe for a continuation of his stuttering behaviors. Several commonplace conditions concerning children who show signs of incipient stuttering should be kept in mind.

> Speech disfluencies are often observed among young children, even among those who are not thought of as children who stutter.

Children can be markedly disfluent without being aware of it.

Increased awareness of disfluency may increase the amount of disfluency.

Speech fluency can be altered both favorably and unfavorably by environmental conditions.

Disfluencies are more likely to become a permanent part of a child's speech if he reacts to them unfavorably.

Direct treatment of the disfluencies may result in increased awareness and increased disfluency and does not guarantee a reduction of disfluency.

### Disfluencies and Their Significance

The amount of disfluency in a child's speech can be observed and measured. The interpretation of the significance of the amount of disfluency present, however, is not an easy matter. There are many ways in which fluent speech may be temporarily interrupted. Some, but not all, of these disruptions of fluency seem to be characteristic of the problem called stuttering.

Metraux, (17) in her interesting account of the speech profiles of preschool children, reports that at the age of 18 months children repeat syllables or words more frequently than not. "The repetition is easy, unforced repetition which can be terminated by himself or by the response of others." The 24-month-old child may repeat "a" before framing his answers to comprehension questions. There is occasional syllable repetition such as "wi-wi-wipe my hands," or "nuh-nuh-ball." "The most common characteristic of repetition at this age is the kind of compulsive repetition of a word or phrase. There is sometimes a variation in the phrase, but it seems necessary to the child to repeat it. With some children the compulsion continues to six or seven repetitions, with others perhaps only twice. Thus a child will say, 'here goes, here goes, here goes,' or 'a ball, dis a ball, dis a ball, Mom.' "

At 36 months, Metraux reports, most children are on an easy repetitive basis with none of the compulsions noted above. When the child does not know the answer, he will ask the question antiphonally with the examiner until she changes the question. Occasionally one hears repetition of the beginning syllable and an [ʌ] or [ʌm] is often used as a starter for speech. "There are some instances of medial repetition as 'the kitty rides in-in-in-that,' but a tonic block on a beginning syllable as 'I wuh———want that doll,' is quite infrequent."

At 42 months repetitions are frequent and occur with almost every child. These repetitions have a somewhat compulsive quality as at 30 months; but at 30 months one can often break the repetition by introducing a new subject or object. At 42 months the repetition often seems to be related to another person, in demand for attention, information, or encouragement so that if one answers him or repeats the same phrase back to him the repetition is usually broken and the child continues his activity, though he may have to complete the cycle and repeat just once more what he has been saying.

Davis (7, 8) studied 62 nonstuttering preschoolers, aged two to five. She found that these children averaged 49 repetitions per 1000 words. She concluded that even if one word in four is a repeated word, either in part or in whole, in a word or phrase repetition, the child is not presenting any abnormality in his speech. She further points out that syllable repetitions were the best measure for determining the children who deviate markedly from the group. Egland (9) compared disfluencies of 26 nonstuttering kindergarten children with the disfluencies of three preschool age stutterers. The nonstuttering group repeated sounds or syllables more often than words or phrases. The speech of the nonstutterer contained a higher percentage of "stalls" ("ah," "um," etc.,) than did the speech samples of the stutterers. The speech of the stutterers had a greater percentage of prolongations.

In studies conducted at the University of Iowa, concerned with the onset of stuttering(15), the great majority of the 246 children considered to be stuttering by their parents repeated sounds, words, or phrases when their parents first looked upon them as stutterers. Approximately three-fourths of the parents did not indicate that the children were doing anything else that they regarded as stuttering other than repeating, except for a few who also said "uh-uh" or "well-uh."

When the children in the experimental group were compared with a matching group of children whose parents did not view them as stutterers, there was not a significant group difference for word repetitions, and significantly more control group children repeated phrases, whereas significantly more experimental group children were reported to repeat sounds or syllables.

To further complicate the problem of deciding whether or not a child stutters, several studies have indicated that agreement, even among trained speech pathologists, is far from perfect. When selecting samples of stuttering from recorded samples of speech, simple modifications in the instructions for observation affect the number of samples of speech designated as "stuttering." For example, Tuthill (18), in one of the earlier studies of this type, instructed his subjects to indicate instances of stuttering as they listened to recordings. He found that many of the samples labeled as "stuttering" were drawn from the speech of persons who did not stutter. Boehmler (6) in a similar study reported that the label "stuttering" was applied more frequently to samples taken from the speech of stutterers than to those taken from the speech of nonstutterers. Both Tuthill and Boehmler found that persons trained in speech pathology were more likely to label a sample of stuttered speech as stuttering than untrained listeners. Williams and Kent (23), however, asked college students to classify speech interruptions as "normal" or "stuttered" and found that many listeners reversed their ratings according to what they were instructed to listen for. If asked to note all instances of "normal" interruptions, they frequently listed the same interruption which they previously had listed as an example of a "stuttered" interruption.

One clue to help distinguish stuttering speech from nonstuttering speech that has been fairly consistent from study to study concerns the type of interruptions or disfluencies. Several studies (7,8,9) have indicated that repetitions of sounds or syllables and prolongations of sounds are more likely to be called "stuttering" than are other types of disfluencies such as revisions or interjections. In other words, there are many ways in which speech can be disfluent, but only certain kinds of disfluencies seem to be a characteristic part of the problem called stuttering. The studies completed on the fluency of speech have not shown that the difference between stutterers and nonstutterers can be made on the basis of how disfluent the speech is. Rather, they have shown us that a large number of the children whose speech was viewed as stuttered speech contained prolongations and that those children did their repeating more on sounds and monosyllables than on words and phrases.

To return to our original problem—when is it proper to classify speech as stuttering? Obviously, as indicated by the preceding information, a child's speech cannot properly be classified as stuttering simply because he is disfluent. Evidently, the type of disfluency he exhibits is important. The greater the number of repetitions and prolongations of single sounds or syllables, the more confidently we can apply the label "stuttered" to his speech.

For the therapist it probably does not matter greatly whether the child's speech is actually more disfluent than normal or the product of exaggerated parental concern, for when the parents become concerned about their child's hesitations and repetitions, the means for reducing the problem are the same in either case. In both cases an attempt is made to provide an attitudinal climate in which concern about the stuttering is not encouraged to flourish. As will be noted in Chapter Three, the type of help given to parents is the same regardless of whether their child's disfluencies are within a so-called normal range or not.

### Differentiating Developmental Stages of Stuttering

A description of overt stuttering characteristics must include an analysis of the severity of the symptoms on display and the particular stage of development of the problem. We want to know not only whether a child stutters, but, if he does stutter, how far the condition has progressed. Any distinction we make between developmental stages of the problem is based on an underlying assumption that different treatments should be applied to stutterers at different stages. Bluemel in 1932 introduced the terms *primary* and *secondary* stuttering to differentiate between the symptoms commonly displayed by stutterers when they were beginning to stutter and the symptoms of stuttering in its advanced form. Primary stuttering was defined as ". . . a simple disturbance of speech in which a delay ensues between the commencement and completion of a word." Secondary stuttering was defined as ". . . consciousness of the defect and attempts to control and conceal it, employing starters, synonyms, etc.," (5). Van Riper expanded these definitions and through his extensive publications helped to popularize these terms. In 1954 (20) he introduced the term "transitional stuttering" to describe more fully the development of primary stuttering as it changes to secondary stuttering.

In 1942 Johnson pointed out that it was difficult to differentiate on the basis of the amount and kind of fluency between the speech of children who are judged by their parents to be stutterers and the speech of children who are not so judged by their parents. In 1953 Glasner and Vermilyea (10) questioned 171 therapists and found a wide range of usages for the term *primary stuttering*. Although many speech therapists referred to the term *awareness* as being crucial, no criteria to measure awareness were presented. Many of them described primary stuttering, however, in terms of repetitions, hesitations, and prolongations but without presenting fluency norms.

Bloodstein, basing his findings on the records of 418 stutterers, concluded, for convenience in classification, that stuttering could be regarded as passing through four major phases in the course of its development. After carefully pointing out that the development of stuttering is actually a continual process of which any sharp definition into phases does some violence, he adds, "The points at which this process has been conveniently arrested are not wholly arbitrary. They represent certain familiar clinical types, each of which is frequently encountered in clinical management." (3:366)*

These diagnostic categories provide for a systematic means of evaluating how far a given child's problem has advanced; these phases emphasize the development of stuttering from its beginning stages to stuttering in its most severe form. Moreover, they help to provide clues to suitable therapy programs.†

A description of Bloodstein's categories is summarized on pp. 20-21. It is readily apparent that the criteria for placing a child in a particular phase include an analysis of both his overt speech characteristics and the reactions he has to speaking. (See especially columns D, E, and H.) The authors have used this four-phase classification system to describe therapy procedures for stutterers and have added the descriptive adjectives *incipient, transitional, confirmed,* and *advanced* to further describe these developmental stages. A summary of the approximate age of onset of these developmental phases of stuttering can be found on page 20.

### A Diagnostic and Evaluative Check List

To illustrate a means of reporting the pertinent findings of an examination of a stutterer, a *Diagnostic and Evaluative Check list* is

---

* The reference number precedes the colon; the page number follows it.

† The authors are indebted to Dr. Bloodstein for his permission to quote these reports extensively. Because this material has been condensed, the reader will find it helpful to consult the original articles on which these statements are based.

| | A. *Clonic Elements* (Repetitions) | B. *Tonic Elements* (Hard Contacts and Prolongations) | C. *Fluent Periods* | D. *Difficult Situations* |
|---|---|---|---|---|
| *Phase 1* (Incipient) | Repetitions of syllables and monosyllables are characteristic symptoms of this phase. | Hard contacts not uncommon but clonic elements predominate. | Usually episodic. Stuttering fluctuates more widely than in any other phase. | Stuttering is intensified by variable sources of communicative pressure. The child is likely to have his greatest difficulty when excited or telling a long story. |
| *Phase 2* (Transitional) | Repetition, hard contact, or associated mannerisms may be dominating symptoms. | See Column A. | Essentially chronic. May disappear briefly but no longer comes in discrete episodes. | (* Distinguishing feature of Phase 2.) Stutters primarily when he talks fast and gets excited. Stutters about equally at home, at school, or with friends. |
| *Phase 3* (Confirmed) | (* Outstanding characteristic of Phase 3.) Fully developed stuttering without avoidance of speech. | See Column A. | Chronic. | Distinctly more difficulty in some situations than in others, and is well aware of these difficult situations. |
| *Phase 4* (Advanced) | See Column F. | See Column F. | Chronic. | Vivid and continual anticipation of stuttering. |

Based on three articles by Oliver Bloodstein in *Journal of Speech and Hearing Disorders*, "The Development of Stuttering: I. Changes in Nine Basic Features, II. Developmental Phases, III. Theoretical and Clinical Implications. 25, 1960, 219-237; 25, 1960, 366-376; 26, 1961, 67-82.

included (Appendix A). This check list focuses the examiner's attention on overt speech patterns. Information concerning interviews with parents of a child who is suspected of beginning to stutter

MOST COMMON AGE OF ONSET OF BLOODSTEIN'S
DEVELOPMENTAL PHASES OF STUTTERING

| *Developmental Phase* | *Approximate Age* |
|---|---|
| One | Preschool |
| Two | Early Elementary School |
| Three | Junior High and High School |
| Four | High School and Older |

will be found in Chapter Three. The importance of the teacher of the stuttering child as a source of cogent information is discussed in Chapter Eight.

| E. *Awareness* | F. *Types of Words Stuttered* | G. *Associated or Secondary Symptoms* | H. *Emotionality and Avoidance* |
|---|---|---|---|
| Does not react emotionally to himself as a stutterer. | Stutterings tend to occur on initial word of sentence and on "small" words such as conjunctions, prepositions, and pronouns. | Not uncommon but clonic elements predominate. | Child generally does not react emotionally as a stutterer and speaks freely in all situations. Essentially no fear or embarrassment. |
| Thinks of himself as a stutterer, but continues to talk freely in all situations. | The stutterings have attached themselves to major parts of speech. | See Column A. | Little or no concern about his stuttering except in severe cases or at moments of unusual difficulty. |
| Is well aware of it and acknowledges it as a personal shortcoming, even —in principle—a problem. | In most cases word substitutions, word and sound difficulties, and, to a lesser degree, conscious anticipations are present at some time during this phase. | Elaborately developed symptomatology with postponement, starting, and release devices. | Dominant reaction to his stuttering when he becomes badly blocked is likely to be exasperation, annoyance or disgust. Essentially no tendency to avoid speaking nor any outward appearance of being troubled by fear or deep embarrassment. |
| Viewed by possessor as serious personal problem. | Special difficulty in response to various sounds, words, situations, and listeners. | Fully developed symptomatology with avoidance, postponement, starting and release devices. | Definite emotional reactions to stuttering—avoidance of certain speaking situations, and evidences of fear and embarrassment. |

* Chief feature distinguishing given phase from next lower phase.

## Fluent Periods

Incipient stuttering fluctuates considerably. Periods of days, weeks, and months may go by without the appearance of an unusual amount of stuttering. Sometimes the stuttering is reported to disappear completely before reappearing (2). More rarely, instances of periods of a year or more of fluency may be reported. Gradually (and the periods of time necessary for these changes to occur varies considerably) the periods of fluency become shorter and shorter and the presence of stuttering is noted more than its absence. It is noteworthy that at the onset of stuttering the disorder is essentially episodic—shifting to essentially chronic and finally to chronic insofar as observable periods of fluency are concerned.

## Awareness or Emotionality

Children who are suspected of being beginning stutterers show little awareness that their speech is different—at least they rarely react emotionally to the way they talk. But, as stuttering becomes an established way of talking, they tend to react more and more emotionally to their way of talking, either inwardly or outwardly, or both. Berry and Eisenson lend support to the importance of measuring reactions to stuttering by pointing out the extreme difference found in some stutterers between the overt symptoms and the person's reactions. After illustrating a case where the observable speech difference far exceeded the speaker's apparent awareness of it, they illustrate the opposite extreme as follows:

> Most speech clinicians will at some time in their careers meet an individual who thinks of himself as a stutterer, but who shows few overt manifestations of stuttering behavior. There is little nonfluency, with only occasional repetition or blocking. There are no apparent tics or grimacings. What the clinician hears and sees appears to be normal and acceptable speech. And yet the speaker himself insists that he is a stutterer and wants to be helped. Stuttering, we might conclude tentatively, has both external and internal aspects. Subjective evaluations as well as the evaluations of other persons become involved in our concepts of stuttering, and in our decisions as to who is to be considered a stutterer and when. (1:249)

A child may react to his disfluencies in many ways. He may feel temporarily frustrated or irritated when he has difficulty saying a word smoothly and quickly, much as he might feel about himself when he stumbles while trying to run up a flight of stairs. At the other extreme, a child may be so sensitive about his stuttering that he refuses to talk for fear of stuttering.

Although some measures of the degree of awareness and emotionality of the child toward his speech disfluency can be made directly by listening to his comments about speech blockings, a considerable portion of our information will come from indirect measures. For example, if a child is observed to avoid the use of a word directly or to show anticipation of speaking difficulty in some other manner, it can be assumed that he does have some degree of negative feelings about making his speech "mistakes." Part of the evaluation of reactions to the stuttering, therefore, concentrates upon measuring the tendency to avoid stuttering. This will be elaborated upon under the section *Associated Symptoms* later in this chapter.

An excellent diagnostic clue is provided through observation of the child's ability to maintain eye contact. If he is reasonably able to look at his audience while speaking, this behavior may coincide with low-level feelings of concern about his stutterings. Evasion of eye contact may be among the first of the clues that will indicate the onset of embarrassment or other negative reactions to his stutterings.

It is quite probable that the largest portion of the child's negative reactions to his speech difficulty is learned from the reactions of the important adults in his environment. In most cases, of course, the child's parents are the individuals most responsible for his attitudes and feelings. Adverse feelings about speaking can be learned, however, from teachers, relatives, or anyone else for that matter. Regardless of the source, if the germs of insecurity are coming from someone else close to a young child, an accounting of this should be made so that appropriate action can be taken in therapy. The kinds of words that are used by the reporting adults to describe the child's symptoms are important, especially at the suspected onset of stuttering. Special note should be made as to whether a child or his parents refer to these symptoms as stuttering, if the child is very young, or if he himself does not outwardly act as if his disfluencies are unusual.

Needless to say, because the amount of emotion and anxiety experienced by the stutterer and those who observe him is the one ingredient that gets the most attention in or out of therapy, the entire contents of this book touch on it in one way or another.

*Consistency and Adaptation*

Van Riper and Hull (21) around 1934 and Johnson and Knott (11) in 1937 were the first to study the adaptation effect, that is, the decrease in stuttering which tends to occur with the repeated reading of the same passage. Since these first studies, this phenomenon has come to be one of the most frequently studied aspects of stuttering behavior.

Frequent references are made about the adaptation effect as a laboratory model of improvement in stuttering. Van Riper and Hull (21) felt that adaptation curves could reflect therapeutic progress. They speculated that if stutterers improved in their overall ability to adapt to speaking situations, adaptation to a reading situation should show also a gain over that shown at the onset of therapy. Johnson, Darley, and Spriestersbach (13) indicated that the adaptation rate may be looked upon as an index of stuttering severity, that is, a stutterer who improves a great deal after reading a passage several times might be expected to respond to therapy better than a stutterer who shows no reduction of stuttering after several readings.

Another phenomenon useful in diagnosis is the *consistency effect.* This phenomenon is seen in the fact that a stutterer reading a passage several times in succession will stutter in the latter readings as many as two-thirds of the words stuttered in the first reading.

According to Johnson, Darley, and Spriestersbach the more consistency a stutterer shows the more strongly his stuttering is conditioned to the words to which he responds by stuttering. The more strongly conditioned his stuttering is to any particular words, the harder it probably will be for him to reach the point where he no longer stutters in response to that word. Thus, they point out, the consistency index has a practical importance to the degree that it indicates the probable modifiability of the stutterer's tendency to stutter in response to particular cues.

In order to test consistency or adaptation of stuttering in a young child who cannot read or who may misunderstand the examiner's purpose, the child can be requested to repeat a series of short sentences from dictation. After marking the stuttered words, the examiner should repeat these same sentences again. The number *1* written above a word would then indicate that it was stuttered the first repetition from dictation and a *2* would indicate that it was stuttered on the second repetition from dictation as
1, 2   2  1, 2  2
in the following example: *Jack likes to feed the little puppies.*

Bloodstein reported that a total of 14 children between three and six years of age tested by this method showed an unmistakable consistency in the distribution of stuttering from the first to second repetitions. The percentages of consistency ranged from 50 to 100, with a mean of 77.1. These children gave no outward sign of reacting to their manner of speaking and had symptoms which consisted of relatively simple repetitions and prolongations (2).

### Repetitions or Clonic Blocks

Repetitions are probably the most common type of disfluency associated with stuttering, especially during the early phases of its development. It is possible to classify the child's repetitions as either relatively relaxed or associated with some degree of tension. Furthermore, the unit of speech that is involved in the repetition can be observed. An individual may repeat a group of words as in the following example, "There are several . . . (pause) . . . there are several ways to build a house." This type of repetition is often used as a postponement device. A repetition may involve only one sound, as in, "I want to g-g-g-g-go home." Repetitions of single sounds are sometimes called "clonic blocks." It is important to observe the degree of tension accompanying the repetition. There is quite a difference between the easy repetitions which a child may use when he is trying to think of the next word to say and the rapid clonic spasm which is sometimes accompanied by a gradual rise in pitch. It is generally useful, therefore, to rate the severity of the tension accompanying the repetition as well as noting the unit of speech which is repeated.

## Hard Contacts and Prolongations

Repetition of sounds, syllables, and monosyllables are mainly characteristic of Phase One stuttering. In every other phase of stuttering these easy, bouncing repetitions and loose prolongations of syllables and sounds are replaced by increasingly tense and forceful attacks on words. Johnson, in describing a child's growing conviction that talking is a difficult process, says:

> Eventually he becomes hesitant enough in trying to say some things to some people that he holds back so much he has to force himself to go ahead, and this seems to be why he begins to speak with some degree of effort or strain. But to exert this effort he tenses up the muscles of his lips or tongue or throat and when he does this he talks more hesitantly and less smoothly, and with some sense of difficulty, and as a result his doubt and uneasiness increases all the more. As a consequence he becomes more hesitant and holds back still more, and so he forces himself harder to go ahead, and in doing this he tenses his muscles increasingly, so that he speaks still less smoothly and with greater sense of difficulty. (16:139)

Normal speech also requires tension in order to create the proper amount of turbulence, friction, or explosions in the outgoing air streams to make conventional audible speech noises. In normal speech the tension is optimal, the contacts and constrictions are just enough so that the sounds can be heard clearly. The words spoken by a person who has had too much to drink are spoken loosely, with less than optimal tension. The stutterer, as he tenses harder forcing himself to go ahead, creates hard contacts of his speech musculature.

Hard contacts or tonic blocks are characteristics of advanced stages of stuttering, although sometimes they may be observed in the speech of a child just beginning to stutter. The area of radiated tension should be noted, and it should be noted whether the contacts are forceful enough to create tremors.

Some stutterers prolong the initial sounds of words, often continuants such as *s, th,* and *f* or their voiced cognates, before attempting a shift into the remainder of the word. Some employ a prolonged, indeterminate vocalized grunt as they attempt plosives such as *p.* These prolongations may be low-pressure, loose contacts of short duration or strong, forceful attacks lasting several seconds.

This struggling and forcing results not only in tight closures and fixed articulatory positions but also in stuttering tremors. According to Van Riper, "the more tense the stutterer becomes, the tighter the lips are pressed until finally a sudden localized burst of tension sets a tremor into motion."

> . . . the stuttering tremor creates in its possessor a vivid feeling of inability and frustration. He feels blocked. His lips seem locked by some mysterious force over which he has no control. His response to the awareness of the tremor is to increase the tension, which only speeds up the tremor, or to make a sudden jerky movement of the structures involved. If this movement is out of phase with the tremor, he often finds release and the word is uttered. If it is in phase, then he bounces right back into his tremor and the same impasse of self-defeating struggle. (20:330)

### Associated Symptoms

As a child becomes more convinced that he does not talk well, he also does more things when talking that make it difficult for him to talk well. For one thing, his increased awareness that talking is difficult keeps him on the alert for trouble in talking. He begins to tense up, suspecting trouble behind every syllable or word. He begins to look for means to hide or minimize his stutterings. At this time, injunctions by parents and teachers to "slow down" or "think of what you are going to say" serve mainly to reinforce the child's convictions that his speaking requires special controls, but they may also help him to think that somewhere, somehow, a means for alleviating his difficulty is available. A child soon learns that merely slowing down doesn't necessarily help because he may have his worst difficulty when it is important to talk fast. He also finds that he would rather not concentrate on what he is about to say because he is mostly concerned with the possibility of getting stuck. So, he tries out other things to see if he can find a way out of his difficulty. For example, he may anticipate trouble with the word "door." Just as with an actual door that sticks, he may push hard against the *d* in order to get through the word. (This may be the cure for a stuck door, but not always for the *word,* because if he pushes hard with his tongue this will only make the *d* "stick" harder.) He may try to wait for the tension to die down before attempting to say *door,* thus creating awkward pauses in the middle of a sentence, he may give up altogether, or he may try another word, just as he might try a window when confronted with a door which won't open.

He may even back up and try to hit the word *door* with a running start—just as he has seen zealous policemen on television break down a door. He may even try to pretend that he never has trouble with doors and with assumed nonchalance breeze up to the door, and if it doesn't open, affect an air that in effect says, "It is immaterial to me whether the door opens or not."

Early observers of stuttering behavior were prone to classify countless numbers of types of stuttering, justifying their findings on the profuse and diverse associated symptoms found to envelop the advanced stages of stuttering. Fortunately the job for the modern observer is less exacting because of a relatively simple classification system introduced by Van Riper. As early as 1937, Van Riper noted that these symptoms were the result of fear of stuttering: unpleasant reactions which attached themselves to what he termed "Jonah" (or feared) words or situations (19). Thus, *Jonah words* were described as those most frequently associated with past stuttering experiences and *Jonah situations* were those made vivid by social penalties. In order to ward off these Jonahs, Van Riper found that stutterers employed a vast variety of tricks and devices that could be divided conveniently into four main groupings: *avoidance, postponement, starter,* and *antiexpectancy devices.* The Diagnostic and Evaluative Checklist in Appendix A employs these categories of expectancy tricks and devices, with examples. Although not all the possible examples of a given type of behavior are included, several examples of each type of associated behavior are indicated to show the kinds of things the speech clinician should expect to find.

The number and variety of associated symptoms that attach themselves more or less permanently to a child's speech depends on how
successfully they have worked in the past to smooth out his speech,
or how desperate he is to climb over the rough spots in talking.

A Phase Four stutterer may use only a few of these devices, or his
speech may be so encumbered and cluttered by them that little else
remains to be observed. In Phase Four stuttering, most of these devices are habitual and often stereotyped. In Phases Three and Two,
they may be transitory in nature, appearing or disappearing, depending on how much a child may need a particular crutch at a
particular time. Whereas these devices and tricks are seen less often
in Phase One stuttering, sometimes they may be observed in the
speech of children as young as four years old.

Along about the end of Phase Two when a child who stutters
has accumulated enough evidence to satisfy himself that talking is
a hazardous, laborious process with embarrassing consequences, he
begins to accumulate these extra mannerisms, postures, and patterns of speech which permit the generalization that there are about
as many types of stuttering as there are stutterers. But this generalization is valid only from this stage in the development on and only
when a child's concern about the way he talks is desperate enough
for him to experiment conscientiously with his way of talking to
find a way that will help him to keep going. The things he does
now are aimed at making it possible for him to get to the end of
his sentence or thought within a reasonable length of time and without showing too much of the clonic or tonic aspects of his stuttering. He usually wants to appear normal, to hide or disguise his
stuttering, and to meet whatever demands are put on him without
feeling embarrassment or shame. How he meets these needs depends
on what behavior is available to him. His motivations to talk and
to appear normal usually determine the form the experiment in
talking will take.

The frequency with which these tricks or devices are adopted by
children as they learn to stutter can be accounted for mainly because they do provide relief at first, if only temporarily. Late in
Phase Two, a child may find a device that works well for a time,
especially if it distracts him enough from his difficulty to say some
words well. However, if a trick or device works, that is, if it helps
him to feel that he can talk better or easier, he may begin to employ the device at the least sign of trouble. When he does this the

device becomes habitual and it thus loses its value as a distraction. The child may even lose sight of why he used the device in the first place. When this occurs, he feels that something is happening to him—something over which he has no control. The behavior is now habitual and set off by almost any expectancy of stuttering.

The device or trick becomes a part of his pattern of stuttering and every block may be preceded by this habitual mannerism or even a set or series of mannerisms. How a device that is employed to keep from stuttering may become an associated observable symptom of stuttering may be illustrated in this way:

A child may find that a word will come easier for him if he presses a finger hard against his desk top or his leg unobtrusively when attempting a feared word. As long as his speech fears can be allayed every time he presses his fingers this is all he will need to do. But there may come a time when he is rattled, or when it is extremely important for him to speak without stuttering. He may be very tense or distracted. At any rate he presses once and the word doesn't come out. He may have to press two or three times before it will, but eventually, the word is released and because it does come out he attributes the successful performance to the work done by his finger. He now feels that he cannot afford to refrain from jabbing himself with his finger because this is his only assurance that he will be able to say the word. He may even bring the finger motion out in the open where it can be seen by others because the most important thing now is to get through the feared word. One woman got so dependent on this kind of device she finally had to give up talking and carried out her communication needs via pad and pencil because if she tried to talk she violently pounded her black-and-blue thigh with her fist. She had started by unobtrusively pressing her finger against her thigh to get the word out.

Another reason for the frequency of these devices is that if done successfully they need not show. Most of the devices are things that a normal speaker does when speaking normally. A normal speaker may back up and start over when groping for an appropriate word. The normal speaker often finds that he can't quite say what he has in mind and may pause or grunt or say "and ah." The normal speaker may rub his nose to hide his confusion or look into the air as if the answer to his dilemma can be found high overhead. The tricks a stutterer uses are often artfully employed and designed to appear normal. If these symptoms become bizarre, it is only because the device has outworn its usefulness and has become habitual, or because the stutterer himself feels that he will be unable to say certain words without the particular mannerism. Stage and movie portrayals of stutterers sometimes depict the stutterer as employing a whistle as a starter or release device, especially if the stutterer is depicted in a "comedy" role. Few real-life stutterers employ this type of device. The stutterer would certainly not identify himself with the role of a "comical stutterer." However, many of these tricks do appear funny to those who do not understand the stutterer's unique problems.

Many other changes in speech may become a part of the stutterer's speech pattern. The excess tension which leads to a repetition or prolongation may also have its affect upon the stutterer's voice quality, speaking rate, or pitch level. One ten-year-old stutterer with whom we worked developed vocal nodules, apparently due to excess laryngeal tension during his stuttering. Wendahl and Cole (22) found that stutterers were easily differentiated from nonstutterers even when their actual stuttering blocks were removed from the tape recorded samples. The stutterers in their study demonstrated a poorer rate of speech, had more force or strain in their voice, and had less rhythmical speech patterns than did the nonstutterers. In other words, even without the stutterings, the speech pattern was different. All such variations from normal speech should be noted, regardless of whether they appear to be a part of the stuttering pattern.

### Evaluation of Related Factors

Obviously there is much more to the examination of a child who stutters than observing his stuttering and his reactions to it. And, there is much more to the therapy process. In order to help a child modify his speech behavior, we need to know something about his general health, the history of his speech and language development, the history of his acquisition of other skills, and anything else which helps us to know how he came to be the child he is.

The conclusion that a child is a "stutterer" often cannot be reached simply on the basis of what is heard coming out of his mouth during a single examination session. This conclusion sometimes requires several observations.

Certain clues will enable us to decide whether to seek more information. For example, if a mother mentions that her child stutters more when reading aloud, we would then want to know more about her child's ability to read, any special problems he may have had in learning to read, or some of the practices commonly used during his reading classes at his school.

The examiner should learn to depend upon a variety of sources for his information. He can learn about the child's health from the medical report, from his parents, or from the school nurse. He can learn about school problems, if any, from his teacher and his cumulative school record. Although the therapist may not be able to check the reliability of some of these indirect reports, he will find that he can relate and understand better what information he does have from his direct observations of the child if he fully utilizes additional available information from other sources.

Appendix B contains a number of questions to which the therapist should have answers. Some of these questions bear, either directly or indirectly, on the etiology of stuttering. It may be futile to try to find the cause of his stuttering since so often a number of related incidents combine. Their cumulative force may set off the stuttering. Often the combination of forces that originally set off stuttering no longer contributes to the problem at the time the child is seen. However, even though some of these factors may no longer operate, it may prove important to inquire about them. In some families strong beliefs exist about conditions that set off the stuttering. The child sooner or later will hear of them if he hasn't already, and the therapist should know of these beliefs if he can get access to them. He should know about how concerned individual members of his family or his teacher are about his stuttering. How much do the parents want to cooperate? How well can they cooperate? Is the child shy or withdrawn? Does he bite his nails, wet the bed, or walk in his sleep? Some of this information is requested in the General Case History (See Appendix C) which provides a means for obtaining general information about the child's speech, physical development, general health, birth history, etc. By comparing the answers to questions in these two forms, plus other questions and observations, several leads will usually turn up which will require further exploration.

### Summarizing and Reporting the Diagnosis and Evaluation

The chapters concerned with modification procedures contain information which is not included in this chapter but which must be understood before the diagnosis and evaluation are complete. Therapy must be understood so that information can be gathered and so that certain appropriate conclusions can be drawn. Although the therapy should be fitted to the child, not the child to the therapy, the diagnosis and the examination should provide information that will prove useful in therapy. The examiner must draw upon his knowledge of normal speech development, of speech disorders in general, of observations that he has made of other children who stutter, of the therapy process, etc. With certain key questions in mind, the examiner will be able to come to a reasonable understanding of the child and his problem. He starts with clues and key pieces of information and fits these parts together to arrive at the imperfect idea of what form the treatment should take. Even then, as he finds out more about a child, he finds he has many unanswered questions and many areas of uncertainty that need clarification.

But decisions need to be made. In spite of the examiner's remaining questions, he is far better able to make a realistic decision about therapy after a systematic appraisal than when he started. He has much more information at his fingertips than he did before he had an opportunity to observe the child closely. As mentioned in Chapter I, there are areas of uncertainty in everything we do. And there will be areas of uncertainty here. But the uncertainty is reduced considerably by the findings obtained from the examination procedure.

After the therapist has collected his information, he should summarize his findings, draw his conclusions, and make his recommendations concerning the treatment to be followed. This is crucial. While the examination is in progress, the act of making a decision can and should be delayed. But when the examination is over, the time to reach conclusions and make recommendations has arrived; it can no longer be postponed.

1. First of all, after reviewing available information, the examiner estimates the relative stage of development of the stuttering; for example, he may decide that the child has reached **Phase Two**, or that he is really not stuttering at all.
2. He then considers recommended treatment procedures for that phase of stuttering. For example, the Phase Two stutterer needs to change some basic evaluations about himself as a speaker.
3. Next, related problems and conditions affecting the child are con-

sidered. He thinks about possibly detrimental attitudes the child or his parents may have; he remembers the sibling in the home who creates additional pressure by his aggressive speech behavior; and he tries to fit these somewhere in the therapy planning.

4. With all this in mind, general plans are laid out of what can and should be attempted during the therapy program.
5. Now the therapist must realize that for the present he need concentrate only on the beginning of the therapy program, and so he considers which of several goals can be aimed at immediately.
6. Decisions are then made on the exact recommendations for the immediate situation. Further observations of the parents and child will modify the original over-all plan, but if these planning steps have been followed carefully the clinician is assured that the treatment program will increase the child's chances of changing his speech behavior for the better.

It is important that the examiner transmit his opinions to those most concerned with the child's problems. Although this may be done either by direct conferences or in written form, it is much better to use the oral report first whenever possible. No matter how well a written report is phrased, there is much less chance for misunderstanding to occur in an oral report. During conversations with a child's parents or his teacher their apprehensions, misunderstandings, conflicts, and objections can be better recognized and coped with. During this kind of reporting, additions, subtractions, and necessary modifications in the information to be presented can be made immediately as the conference develops. When therapy steps are to be initiated, it is important that the parent or teacher thoroughly understand the why, what, and how of therapy. Sometimes it is more difficult to justify indirect therapy to a parent than it is to explain that direct measures are needed. Parents are accustomed to having their child's problems solved by having something done—something concrete, such as administering a pill or an injection, which makes little demand for changes in their own behavior. Indirect therapy often places considerable demands upon the parents and the teacher. They must know reasonably well what will be required of them and why.

Even if it is found that a child's speech is normal, it is not enough simply to tell his parents or teacher this. If parents or teachers feel that something is wrong, then the therapist should continue the conferences until he feels that he knows what their concern is and that they completely understand why he arrived at his conclusions. The therapist should continually check and recheck to make certain that parents and teachers understand. Real communication must take place, and this is rarely an easy accomplishment.

Reporting examination results must not be overlooked or underestimated in importance. The manner in which the results are transmitted to the parents probably affects very greatly how they will react to the child and his stuttering.

The therapy process doesn't really start with the clinician's decision to start therapy. So far as the child is concerned, the therapist's attitude, his special knowledge, his insights, and the way he reacts to the child's stuttering have an impact on the child and his frame of mind. Indeed, therapy has started during the diagnosis even though the first "therapy session" may not yet have been scheduled.

*References*

1. BERRY, M. F. and J. EISENSON. *Speech Disorders: Principles and Practices of Therapy* (New York: Appleton-Century-Crofts, 1956).
2. BLOODSTEIN, O. "The Development of Stuttering: I—Changes in Nine Basic Features," *Journal of Speech and Hearing Disorders,* XXV (1960), 219-37.
3. ————. "The Development of Stuttering: II—Developmental Phases," *Journal of Speech and Hearing Disorders,* XXV (1960), 366-76.
4. ————. "The Development of Stuttering: III—Theoretical and Clinical Implications," *Journal of Speech and Hearing Disorders,* XXVI (1961), 67-82.
5. BLUEMEL, C. S. "Primary and Secondary Stammering," *Quarterly Journal of Speech,* XVIII (1932), 187-200.
6. BOEHMLER, R. M. "Listener Responses to Non-Fluencies," *Journal of Speech and Hearing Research,* I (1958), 132-41.
7. DAVIS, D. M. "The Relation of Repetitions in the Speech of Young Children to Certain Measures of Language Maturity and Situational Factors: Part I," *Journal of Speech Disorders,* IV (1939), 303-18.
8. ————. "The Relation of Repetitions in the Speech of Young Children to Certain Measures of Language Maturity and Situational Factors: Parts II and III," *Journal of Speech Disorders,* V (1940), 235-46.
9. EGLAND, G. O. "Repetitions and Prolongations in the Speech of Stuttering and Nonstuttering Children," In *Stuttering in Children and Adults,* W. Johnson and R. R. Leutenegger (eds.) (Minneapolis: University of Minnesota Press, 1955).
10. GLASNER, P. J. and F. D. VERMILYEA. "An Investigation of the Definition and Use of the Diagnosis, "Primary Stuttering,'" *Journal of Speech and Hearing Disorders,* XVIII (1953), 161-67.
11. JOHNSON, W. and J. R. KNOTT. "Studies in the Psychology of Stuttering: I—The Distribution of Moments of Stuttering in Successive Read-

ings of the Same Material," *Journal of Speech Disorders,* II (1937), 17-19.
12. ———, *et al.* "A Study of the Onset and Development of Stuttering," *Journal of Speech Disorders,* VII (1942), 251-57.
13. ———, F. DARLEY, and D. C. SPRIESTERSBACH. *Diagnostic Manual in Speech Correction* (New York: Harper & Row, Publishers, 1952).
14. ———*et al. Speech Handicapped School Children* (rev. ed.), (New York: Harper & Row, Publishers, 1956).
15. ———, and associates. *The Onset of Stuttering* (Minneapolis: University of Minnesota Press, 1959).
16. ———. *Stuttering and What You Can Do About It* (Minneapolis: University of Minnesota Press, 1961).
17. METRAUX, R. W. "Speech Profiles of the Pre-School Child 18 to 54 Months," *Journal of Speech and Hearing Disorders,* XV (1950), 37-53.
18. TUTHILL, C. E. "A Quantitative Study of Extensional Meaning with Special Reference to Stuttering," *Speech Monographs,* XIII (1946), 81-98.
19. VAN RIPER, C. "The Growth of the Stuttering Spasm," *Quarterly Journal of Speech,* XXIII (1937), 70-73.
20. ———. *Speech Correction: Principles and Methods,* Fourth Ed. (Englewood Cliffs, N.J.: Prentice-Hall, Inc., 1963).
21. ———, and C. J. HULL. "The Quantitative Measurement of the Effect of Certain Situations on Stuttering," In *Stuttering in Children and Adults,* W. Johnson and R. R. Leutenegger (eds.) (Minneapolis: University of Minnesota Press, 1955).
22. WENDAHL, R. W., and J. COLE. "Identification of Stuttering During Relatively Fluent Speech," *Journal of Speech and Hearing Research,* IV (1961), 281-86.
23. WILLIAMS, D. E., and L. R. KENT. "Listener Evaluations of Speech Interruptions," *Journal of Speech and Hearing Research,* I (1958), 124-31.

*Chapter Three*

The Modification of Incipient
Stuttering (Phase One)

*In this first developmental phase of the disorder the difficulty is not present consistently; it comes and goes. The child's stutterings consist mainly of repetitions of syllables and monosyllabic words. Stuttering tends to occur on the initial word of the sentence and small relational words. Stuttering is intensified by variable sources of communicative pressure. Generally speaking, the child does not react to himself emotionally as a stutterer, speaks freely in all situations, and has essentially no fear or embarrassment. Although environmental or indirect therapy plays a role in treatment at all developmental levels of stuttering, it is discussed in detail in this chapter as a major approach to the modification of Phase One stuttering.*

When a child begins to stutter, or show signs of beginning to stutter, the prognosis for improvement is as good as it will ever be. Stuttered speech is not a problem only because the possessor's speech is marred. Stuttered speech becomes a problem only when someone is concerned that it is a problem, whether it be the child, his parents, or someone else. At the onset of stuttering, one of the important considerations is not so much *is the child really stuttering* as it is *is the child himself, or important members of his audience, concerned about the way he talks?*

To modify or eliminate the problem, it is necessary to determine who is concerned, why the person or persons are concerned, and if the source of concern can be altered or eliminated. The preceding chapter discussed some of the ways for determining whether the child, or his parents, or both, show concern. Why a person is concerned is less easy to determine. The basis for concern may spring from a variety of sources.

The frequency of observed stutterings or stuttering-like behaviors may, indeed, be unusually high or thought to be unusually high.

Stuttering may have been present somewhere in the family line.

An important adult in the family may have a vivid unpleasant memory of someone who had stuttered severely.

The child may have had an emotional upset accompanied by, or followed by, an increase in disfluency.

The child may be reflecting concern he has observed in others.

His parents may doubt their ability to raise their child properly and the concern over possible indications of stuttering may be part of a generalized concern for the welfare of their child.

Certainly a combination of the reasons listed above could be at the root of the concern, plus many, many others.

Whether the source of concern, that is, the disfluencies, can be dissipated also depends on a variety of circumstances:

If the child stutters because someone has been effective in transmitting wrongly evaluated information about what the child is doing, the success of therapy will depend on whether the persons involved, including the child, can be dissuaded from continuing to so evaluate their perceptions.

If the child is apprehensive about being able to communicate effectively because of personal shortcomings as a talker—aside from his stutterings—the success of therapy will depend on whether his oral communication skills can be improved to a level at which he will consider himself an adequate talker.

If the child is constantly exposed to emotionally upsetting conditions which precipitate his stuttering, the success of therapy will depend on how alterable these conditions are.

If the child is constantly subjected to external communicative stress and pressure which he cannot withstand, success of therapy will depend on whether the circumstances which induce disfluency can be altered sufficiently to allow him to strengthen his oral communication skills, or on whether he can be toughened sufficiently to cope with these pressures.

### Environmental Therapy for Incipient Stuttering

If stuttering is to be kept from developing to a more advanced form, it is important that the child not conclude that talking is an unreasonably difficult thing to do, or, if the idea that talking is difficult has already taken hold, the child should be helped to correct this misconception. This is not an easy correction to make, and several sections of this book are devoted to the means for doing it.

When there is little evidence for believing that a child has reached an unfavorable conclusion about his ability to talk well, there is considerable danger that a course of action aimed directly at showing him what to do or how to talk may increase an only minimal or even latent awareness that he has trouble talking. Simply stated, the reasons for not taking direct action at this time are the same as the reasons given by dentists who recommend that parents not tell a child, just as he is about to climb in the dentist's chair, that it won't hurt. This may give him food for thought that hadn't occurred to him before.

Usually, at this level of development, no attempt is made to work directly on a child's speech if it can be avoided, because it is difficult to know what the child is thinking. Usually he is a young child of preschool or early elementary school age. His ability to verbalize his understanding or insight is limited. It is difficult for a therapist to know how the child evaluates the generalizations and instructions of therapy. He can act out his thoughts, but it is difficult and sometimes risky to try to interpret what his actions mean. Thus, discretion requires that direct confrontation with his stuttering be delayed until other ways of allaying or altering his behavior have been attempted.

Clinical evidence confirms that behind-the-scenes manipulations, usually through a working relationship with the child's parents, help provide a climate favorable to the development of nonstuttered speech. Because this can be done without involving the child directly, it is referred to as *environmental* or *indirect therapy*. Because it precludes the dangers inherent in involving the child directly, it is the safest kind of therapy when the child is considered to be a Phase One stutterer. Following is a discussion of some of the major environmental approaches.

### The Therapist as a Source of Information

One of the best ways the therapist can create changes in a stuttering child's environment is by transmitting reliable, pertinent information on stuttering and on speech and language development to the child's parents and teachers. The kind of information provided and the manner in which it is done will have a significant effect on the attitudes and reactions the parents will have toward the child and his problem. The type of information that should usually be provided will be discussed first.

*Disfluency as a Normal Part of Learning to Talk*

Probably the most significant fact about stuttering which can be presented to the parents is that disfluency is a "normal" phenomenon. Stutterings—at least some forms of speech disruptions—are a normal part of learning to talk. Stutterings such as hesitations, repetitions, and retrials are commonly observed in the speech of many young children, and they may be symptomatic only of a child's efforts to learn to speak properly. Van Riper mentions the following counterpressures to normal fluent speech which affect the speech of normal speakers as well as those whose speech is viewed as stuttered.

> 1. *Inability to find or remember the appropriate words.* "I'm thinking of- of- of- of- uh- that fellow who- uh—oh yes, Aaronson. That's his name." This is the adult form. In a child it might occur as: "Mummy, there's a birdy out there in the . . . in the . . . uh . . . he's . . . uh . . . he . . . he . . . he wash his bottom in the dirt." Similar sources of hesitant speech are found in bilingual conflicts, where vocabulary is deficient; in aphasia; and under emo-

tional speech exhibition, as when children forget their "pieces."
_2. Inability to pronounce or doubt of ability to articulate._ Adult
form: "I can never say 'sus-stus-susiss-stuh-stuhstiss—oh, you know
what I mean, figures, statistics." The child's form could be illustrated
by "Mummy, we saw two poss-poss- uh- possumusses at the zoo. Huh?
Yeah, two puh-possums." Tongue twisters, unfamiliar sounds or
words, too fast a rate of utterance, and articulation disorders can
produce these sources of speech hesitancy.

_3. Fear of the unpleasant consequences of the communication._
"Y-yes, I-I-I- uh I- t-took the money." "W-wi-will y- you marry m-me?"
"Duh-don't s-s-spank me Mum-mummy." Some of the conflict may
be due to uncertainty as to whether the content of the communication is acceptable or not. Contradicting, confessing, asking favors,
refusing requests, shocking, tentative vulgarity, fear of exposing
social inadequacy, fear of social penalty in school recitations or
recitals.

_4. The communication itself is unpleasant, in that it recreates an_
_unpleasant experience._ "I cu-cu-cut my f-f-f-finger, . . . awful bi-big
hole in it." "And then he said to me, 'You're fi-f-f-fired.'" The narra-
tion of injuries, injustices, penalties often produces speech hesitancy.
Compulsory speech can also interrupt fluency.

_5. Presence, threat, or fear of interruption._ This is one of the
most common of all the sources of speech hesitancy. Incomplete
utterances are always frustrating and the average speaker always
tries to forestall or reject an approaching interruption. This he
does by speeding up the rate, filling in the necessary pauses with
repeated syllables or grunts or braying. This could be called "fili-
bustering," since it is a device to hold the floor. When speech becomes a battleground for competing egos, this desire for dominance
may become tremendous. More hesitations are always shown in
attempting to interrupt another's speech as well as in refusing
interruption.

_6. Loss of the listener's attention._ Communication involves both
speaker and listener, and when the latter's attention wanders or is
shifted to other concerns, a fundamental conflict occurs ("Should I
continue talking . . . even though she isn't listening? If I do, she'll
miss what I just said. . . . If I don't, I won't get it said. Probably
never . . . Shall I? . . . Shan't I?") The speaker often resolves
this conflict by repeating or hesitating until the speech is very
productive of speech hesitancy. "Mummy, I-I-I- want a . . .
Mummy, I . . . M . . . Mumm . . . Mummy, I . . . I want a
cookie." Disturbing noises, the loss of the listener's eye contact,
and many other similar disturbances can produce this type of fluency interrupter (11:365-66).

These communicative pressures should be discussed in the light
of their possible contribution to "normal" disfluency. It should be

pointed out, however, that when a child is temporarily insecure, tired, restless, excited, or confused, counterpressures of this sort may temporarily increase the frequency of disfluencies. If the child is generally insecure or in a state of prolonged tension because of poor health, unsuccessful performance in school subjects, unequal competition for affection, or for any of a number of other reasons, disfluencies may appear to be a regular feature of the child's pattern of speech. Normality in this case means that the disfluencies can be accounted for, not because the child "has something," but because of a "normal" reaction to things happening to him.

Another reason for presenting information of this kind is to prevent indiscriminate lumping of all kinds of disfluency under one heading. Discussion should help lead to a calm appraisal of the child's disfluency. If important adults look on his stuttering as a dreaded affliction, they should be helped toward a more perceptive view of stuttering in which they look on the phenomenon with interest instead of awe.

## The Development of Stuttering

It is sometimes helpful to describe the typical pattern of stuttering as it appears at the onset and to contrast it with more advanced forms. This emphasizes the urgency of keeping the disfluency from changing to a more acute form. Usually parents are already impressed with the possibility that the stutterings may change to a more advanced form, but, whenever strong resistance is encountered to suggested changes in attitudes or management techniques, a presentation of developmental facts may be the only way to shake these convictions.

> In Billy's case, both of his parents agreed wholeheartedly that it would be better to change their pattern of living than his pattern of speech. Where father had held long animated conversations with him upon his return from work, strongly urging him to tell him all about what he had done during the day, he now is quite content to let Billy talk if he wishes—and he listens to him when he talks.
>
> Mother now assigns him more responsibilities around the house, in marked contrast to her previous reluctance to trust him to do anything, and she also lets him visit the neighborhood playground occasionally with the neighbor's children—without her. Instead of vigorous romps and strenuous games of hide-and-seek—with father jumping out from behind doors—to Billy's excited delight, father now reads quietly to him in the evening.

Grandfather, who also lives with them, thought it was all a lot of nonsense until we invited him to the college clinic. He insisted, "If the boy would just think of what he wanted to say, he wouldn't have any trouble." We hooked grandfather up to the delayed sidetone recorder and asked him to simply think of what he wanted to say as he talked into the microphone. Although we assured him that it wasn't the same thing that was happening to Billy when he talked, Grandfather said, "I guess there is more to this than I had thought." After he sat in on a therapy session with a group of teen-age stutterers he said to the therapist who had been working with Billy's parents, "Now tell me what I should do to help; I've learned my lesson."

The therapist should explain to the parents that the child's concept of himself as a speaker may change adversely if more severe stuttering symptoms should appear. The therapist should emphasize that the possibility of "becoming afraid to speak" is a much more serious problem for the child than not being able to speak fluently. Unless they clearly understand this important fact, they may continue reacting to the child's stutterings in ways which will increase rather than decrease his problem.

## Misconceptions about Stuttering

In many cases, it helps to discuss some of the more common misconceptions about stuttering with the parents and teachers. They may be helped by knowing that their child is probably not tongue-tied and not necessarily emotionally disturbed or mentally retarded. It is often wise to mention that stuttering is apparently not a matter of "thinking faster than one speaks" or "speaking faster than one thinks" or even of "not thinking of what one is going to say."

The examples of misconceptions we have heard over the years would make a truly amusing list to read, were it not for the fact that every misconception leads to inappropriate and sometimes even damaging attempts to cure the problem. Among our cases, stuttering has been attributed to eating dill pickles (especially during a full moon or during menstruation), drinking chocolate sodas, being tickled, and of course, the proverbial tongue-tie and pinched nerve.

One child we knew had his tongue clipped four times. His parents had taken him to a rural "doctor" because he was tongue-tied. The treatment of choice was to clip the tongue, even though the judgment of the child's being tongue-tied was reached on the basis of listening to the child's speech errors and not by examining the frenum of the tongue or measuring the mobility of the tongue tip. Since the child's speech symptoms persisted after each tongue clipping the process was repeated.

So long as parents are bound by such misconceptions, not only are they likely to react inappropriately but they will be inclined to resist efforts to find reasonable causes for the child's excess tension. As mentioned elsewhere in this chapter, however, the therapist will be wise to tread cautiously when seeking to rid someone of a belief firmly held.

## *The Why of Stuttering*

Most parents will want to know why their child has a problem. In most cases the therapist will be unable to give a definite answer. It may be wise to mention briefly the three main groups of theories; that is, (a) that stuttering is due to a physical difference: (b) that stuttering is due to psychological differences; or (c) that stuttering is learned behavior. The wise therapist will hasten to add that at present the available evidence does not clearly favor any one of the three theories and will indicate to the parent that the best approach is to continue to observe their child carefully and to attempt some modifications of factors which possibly affect the child's speech behavior. Energies can be expended more profitably than by worrying unduly about what *caused* stuttering. Encourage these parents to modify the problem in the direction of less anxiety both for themselves and their child.

## *Speech and Language Development*

In addition to giving the parents information about stuttering in particular, it is usually helpful to increase their understanding of speech and language development in general. This type of information may be as valuable in modifying their reactions as is the information on stuttering itself. For example, the parent who expects a child to have better articulation than should be expected for his age may tend to place undue pressure on the child to be fluent. The available facts concerning the development of articulatory ability can be discussed and reference made, if necessary, to normative studies such as Poole's research on the chronological order of maturation of consonant speech sounds(7). The therapist should explain something about the difficulties a child normally encounters as he attempts to learn our language code. In this explanation, the therapist may emphasize that the child has probably already acquired the most important aspects of the code system; that is, he has learned well the intricacies of speaking our language.

In explaining the process of language development, the therapist should point out that the emotional value of language is no less important than the ideational value. Speech is useful not only for conveying facts, but also for communicating feelings—both good and bad. This paragraph from a booklet on the prevention of stuttering illustrates the importance of the emotional aspects of speech development:

> But speech is also the way we blow off steam, vent the emotional acids. Many of us falter in this expression. Many of us never learn the magical power of speech to deal with emotion. Many little children, otherwise fairly fluent, find their mouths stumbling when their anxieties, hostilities, or guilt feeling cannot be bottled up another little moment. The mouth is the vent of vents. Let us show our children that they can ease themselves by opening their mouths and letting the evils come out in words, that we ˙can bear them, that we can even share them. Troubles shared are thereby halved, whittled down to bearable size. By transforming the roily squirting of the glands into the magic of words do we become more able to handle the bitter stuff. If we can help our children learn to handle their emotions, we have given them new powers which can stand them in good stead all the rest of the days of their lives (10:23).

And of course, letting off steam is only one segment of emotional communication. The mother's emotion of love is communicated to the child even before he learns to talk. Much of the cooing, gurgling, and babbling which take place between the infant and his parents is emotional communication. This transference of affection is a necessary ingredient in learning to talk. And perhaps as adults we have not lost as much of the emotional motivation for talking as it might seem. The professor who "turns a neat phrase" during his lecture might indeed be saying, "Look at me— See how important I am!" The parent who states, "I just don't know what I'm going to do with Jimmy," might in reality be expressing a feeling of dependence. We express aggressions, hostilities, affection, and even love in much of what passes for "intellectual content." This is a legitimate part of learning to talk.

If possible, it is useful to have parents accompany the therapist in observing the language performance of children of various ages. He can show them how one child misarticulates a number of sounds—how another displays an inability to control his pitch level —how another has difficulty thinking of words to say. Such observa- tions, if properly directed, count more than any words.

One of the best descriptions of the type of information to pre- sent to parents of stutterers is found in the text, *Speech Correction in the Schools,* by Eisenson and Ogilvie. This is the type of infor- mation that is advocated:

1. Every child has his own rate and pattern of language and speech development just as he has his own rate and pattern of physical growth and motor development. A slower than "normal" develop- mental pattern does not necessarily mean that the child is retarded.

2. Language and speech development are related to some factors over which the child has no control. These include the position and number of children in the family, the linguistic ability and intelli- gence of the parents, the child's sex, and the appropriateness of motivation and stimulation for the child to talk. A first child tends to begin to talk earlier than a second, and a second earlier than a third. Girls, by and large, talk earlier and more proficiently than boys. The child who is urged to talk too soon may be more delayed in beginning than the child who begins to talk when he is ready and needs to talk.

3. Attentive and available parents are much more helpful for the development of speech than either anxious or nonavailable parents.

4. Language is not likely to be used unless its use is associated with pleasure.

5. Children should enjoy making sounds before sounds are used as words. Even after children begin to use words they continue to enjoy making sounds when they have nothing to communicate.

6. Many children do not establish sound proficiency until they are almost eight years of age. A young child is entitled to lisp, hesitate, and repeat without being corrected except by good example.

7. Children must hear good speech if they are to become good speakers.

8. Fluency does not become established all at once. Most preschool children are nonfluent some of the time, and many of them are nonfluent much of the time. Nonfluencies up to ten per cent of utterance are not in themselves abnormal.

9. Absence of speech fluency becomes important and a matter for concern when it is associated with specific recurring situations or events. Parents should note whether the child becomes increasingly

nonfluent when frustrated, when fatigued, or when talking to particular persons. If the child's nonfluencies increase sharply in these situations, control of them, if possible, is recommended. Control may take place either by avoiding the situation or by doing nothing that requires the child to communicate in these situations. By communicating we mean having to answer questions that call for precise answers. Nothing, however, should be done to give the child a feeling that he is not to speak if he wishes to do so.

Parents should also note whether the child becomes increasingly nonfluent when he bids or competes for attention. If this is so, then parents should be alert to give the child quick attention when he is normally fluent. This is important so that increased nonfluencies do not result in greater satisfaction than normal fluency (5:219-21).

## *Bibliotherapy*

Below is a selected list of booklets and books written especially for parents who want to know more about stuttering through reading about it. These booklets and books deal mainly with the onset and first stages.

Johnson, Wendell, *Toward Understanding Stuttering.* The National Society for Crippled Children and Adults, Inc., 2023 West Ogden Avenue, Chicago 12, Illinois (1958, 36 pp.).

Johnson, Wendell, *An Open Letter to the Mother of a Stuttering Child.* Interstate Printers and Publishers, Danville, Illinois (1941, 4 pp.).

Johnson, Wendell, *Stuttering and What You Can Do About It.* University of Minnesota Press, Minneapolis (1961, 208 pp.).

Lassers, Leon, *8 Keys to Normal Speech and Child Adjustment.* Speech Aid Series, Leon Lassers, 2855 34th Avenue, San Francisco 16, Calif. (1945, 97 pp.).

Miller, Elvena, *Is Your Child Beginning to Stutter?* Seattle Public Schools, Seattle, Washington (1955, 23 pp.).

Mulder, Robert, *Tangled Tongues: Helping the Stuttering Child.* Educational Materials Productions, Oregon College of Education (1960, 16 pp.).

Pennington, R. Corbin, *For Parents of a Child Beginning to Stutter.* Interstate Printers and Publishers, Danville, Illinois (16 pp.).

*Stuttering: Its Prevention.* Speech Foundation of America, Memphis, Tenn. (1962, 64 pp.).

Van Riper, Charles, *Stuttering.* The National Society for Crippled Children and Adults, Inc., 2023 West Ogden Avenue, Chicago 12, Illinois (1954, 60 pp.).

Van Riper, Charles, *Your Child's Speech Problems.* Harper & Row, Publishers, 49 E. 33rd St., New York 16, N.Y. (1961, 139 pp.).

### The Reception of the Information

The receptiveness of parents to information provided by the therapist may be just as important as the information itself. Some parents will be eager to hear all—others may appear disinterested or even resistant to receiving advice. There are a number of reasons for resistance. Some of the important reasons are discussed in the next several paragraphs.

*Parental Concern*

Speech is a social phenomenon and is closely tied in with parental ego. Most parents derive strong measures of pride in teaching their children to talk. A child's speech acquisition is tied closely to his parents' wish fulfillment and most parents strive diligently to teach their children to talk properly. What happens when a young child is taught to say "bye-bye" may help to illustrate parental ego-involvement. The word *bye-bye* is often taught with a gesture— the child is encouraged to wave his hand while making the appropriate noises. Parents push for this accomplishment as assiduously as they do toilet training; some do this even more so because it is a *public, social* gesture of an accomplishment taught. Some surreptitiously wiggle their infant's elbow to announce their child's entrance into a social speaking world. The ability to speak early is often thought to be an indication of the child's ability to learn and a reflection of the ability of the teacher. This belief is widely held, even though only partly true. But when a child learns to speak well and early, his parents are proud of him (and of themselves). The child is ready to go into the world as a talker, well fitted to represent his family.

Stuttering receives inordinate attention because it is public— it is seen and heard and is not as hideable as is bed wetting, nail biting, negativism, or other foibles encountered in young children. Also, stuttering is often thought of in the public mind as a sign of nervousness. Nervousness though here undefined,* is believed to stem from personal weakness or poor parental management. Because the act of stuttering can reflect unfavorably on the child's parents, they tend to feel vaguely responsible for its occurrence, if they do not feel downright guilty about it. Some parents are un-

---

* Rarely is it defined except vaguely in terms of an undesirable type of behavior.

duly anxious to correct their own real or imagined shortcomings
as revealed by the stuttering.

Certainly, anxiety is also motivated by concern for the child and
his welfare. But the point stressed here is that one of several reasons why parental anxiety is a common concommitant of stuttering
is because stuttering is a public event. People see it and hear it and
it is not something that can remain for very long a family affair
to be coped with in the privacy of the home. Parents are exposed
to the false evaluations of others. They are the recipients of advice
given both tactfully and otherwise. They, along with their child,
are subject to public trial and too often judged guilty of wrong-
doing, without a fair chance to prove their innocence. Some parents
even believe that they are judged fairly and attempt to expiate
their guilt by making it up to the child, protecting him from possible embarrassments, tension, and conflict. Many parents try to lesson their burden of guilt by actively attempting to free their child
from his stutterings. These parents may caution the child to think
of what he is trying to say. They may caution him to slow down,
or to speed up, or may help him by saying certain difficult words
for him. Some try to ignore it, while others find morbid fascination
in the fact that their child has difficulty with certain words or
sounds and do not repress their expression of concern, even in
front of their child. They often do this in the name of self-efface-
ment or bewilderment. "I just don't know what to make of my
child." Some do it for even less plausible and less helpful reasons,
but indicate that it is something that they shouldn't be held ac-
countable for. Some parents try to shame or ridicule stuttering out
of existence. Some try to buy its demise. One third-grade boy was
promised a five-dollar gold piece by his teacher and a new bicycle
by his parents if he would stop his stuttering by the end of the
school year.

Several words of caution are required. Parents, perhaps unknow-
ingly, may be on the defensive about their child's stuttering. They
may have been blamed for their child's behavior. They may think
that they will be in for some more of the same from the speech
therapist. They may feel that no one really understands what their
child is going through—or, for that matter, what they are going
through. A therapist rarely obtains more than an incomplete idea
of what makes up the perceptions of anyone, and this fact prompts

him to contain and hold back his judgments. But what if a parent does show concern and the concern seems to be excessive?

Because a therapist knows the consequences of stuttering he is apt to carry some convictions about it. One of them is that parents tend to get unnecessarily upset about signs of stuttering and thereby contribute to its cause or perpetuation. Some parents do. But there is more to it than that.

Parental concern does not invariably increase stuttering. Little is really known about the other side of this particular coin. Little investigation has been made of those children who are suspected of stuttering but whose stuttering "goes away." Studies which turn up evidence that parents of stutterers are concerned about the way their children talk must also be able to demonstrate that these parents have no reason to be concerned. When stuttering grows and parental concern is also evident, such concern is likely to be called "misguided" and thought to be contributing directly to the problem. But parental concern may even pay off in reduced stuttering. Unquestionably, this avenue of research is relatively inaccessible to quantitative appraisal. But it cannot be denied entirely that the same kinds of pressures may turn away stuttering as well as turn it on.

Reports are heard of stuttering that was "outgrown" or "cured." But when these reports include evidence that bribes, ridicule, shame, strong injunctions to stop stuttering, and the like were used to help it disappear, there is a strong inclination to shrug and conclude that stuttering was not at stake. The child, it is contended, was not really stuttering to begin with.

The reality of "parental concern" is that parents are concerned about those they deeply love. It is easy to debase genuine love by speaking of "love objects," "covert rejection," or "ownership" as if parental love itself was misguided. When stuttering severity and parental concern grow in direct proportion, it is wrong to assume that concern is wrong, or that this display of concern is perverted love, or even that the growth of concern is causing the growth in stuttering. Concern may be a causative factor, but not nearly as often as one would be led to believe.

Parents may wonder if they are overly concerned and even feel guilty about it, but the laws of nature and man provide that they *be* concerned. Concern, whether it be just enough or too much, is a *fact* of parenthood and not something unusual, or abnormal, or misguided. Favorable things can be said about parental concern even though it sometimes backfires. Children turn out right more often than wrong, and most often, the reason children turn out as well as they do is because their parents showed their concern—and even excessively.

Acknowledgment of the legitimacy of a parent's concern is extremely important in staving off defensive rejection of the therapist's efforts. The therapist may need to preface suggestions for covering up reactions of anxiety to a child's stuttering by admitting the natural inclination for being concerned. This caution should extend to reading material recommended to the parent and should lead the therapist to carefully examine bibliotherapy items and to estimate the parent's reaction before suggesting their use.

*Authority*

Certain things about the therapist himself affect the parents' receptivity to what is said about their behavior or that of their child. If a therapist is young and without experience in raising children or teaching them, some parents hesitate to accept him as an "authority." Some parents take a firm "I'm from Missouri—show me!" attitude. The best way to be effective is to go easy. Avoid going further than is necessary. Avoid telling more than needs to be told, or trying to give the impression of considerable experience. The therapist needs to be honest with himself and with the child's parents and with the facts of his experience. Maturity, sincerity, and adequate knowledge about speech and language development should be presented from a "From what I understand" frame of reference. Most parents understand that difficult problems rarely have easy solutions.

The matter of tact when dealing with resistant parents and teachers is obvious. Of foremost importance is a calm recognition by the therapist of the necessity and value of resistance. If the therapist can react to such attitudes without being defensive, he will be in a much better position to focus upon the emotions of the parent and to react to them in such a way as to instill confidence.

One of the best ways the therapist can avoid losing the confidence of parents and teachers is to maintain a realistic evaluation of his own competencies. "Realistic" refers to both strengths and limitations. The therapist should realize that he probably understands more about stuttering and about speech and language development than anyone else concerned with the child. At the same time, he needs to recognize that the parent and the teacher know the child better—know more about how this child will react and has reacted under many different circumstances. Both the parent and teacher certainly have more opportunities to observe the child. Much of our weakness in therapy comes from seeking to overextend our area of competence. More will be said about this later.

Beasley suggests that the therapist view himself less as an authority and more as one who joins parents in seeking a better understanding of the child and how he can be helped. "The therapist reaches out to parents as people who are operating in the best way they know at the moment, who probably have a lowered sense of self-worth because of the difficulties the child is having, and who have need to express their doubts and uncertainties" (1:319). Furthermore, the relationship between the speech therapist and the parent is not essentially different from the relationship between a speech therapist and a child. Beasley says the components of this relationship involve *respect* for the parents' present functioning, *understanding* of their need to preserve their defenses whatever they may be, *acceptance* of the parents as people of worth in their own right, *sensitivity* to parents' feeling of hope and despair, and *compassion* for their situation (1:319).

### Providing Information about Stuttering

The student in speech therapy is keenly aware of the tremendous amount of writing concerned with the problem of stuttering. When seeking to provide information about stuttering to parents, the goals of this educative process must be kept in mind. It is not the therapist's task to give them an abstract of his last college course in stuttering. It is not his job to impress them with his vast store of knowledge. When one visits a dentist with an aching tooth, one does not want to hear all about the anatomy of the mouth nor even about the various techniques of filling a cavity. There are areas of disagreement in dentistry just as there are in stuttering—but the patient does not usually care to know about them. The purpose of informing parents about stuttering is to help them deal adequately with their child's problem. This includes dispelling some of their misconceptions, some of their worries, some of their anxieties. But

too much information may tend to increase anxiety rather than reduce it.

### Provision for a Course of Indirect Action

Environmental therapy can bog down and be resisted or rejected
simply because it does not provide an outlet for a parent's honest
desire to do something concrete for his child. Parents want more
than background information or assurance. They want some "yes"
and "no" answers and they want some specific ways to handle specific situations. It is entirely possible to provide for action without
directly involving the child. For example, probably the most important area of indirect action is concerned with helping parents
react to their child's stutterings and disfluencies so as not to increase
his difficulties. Concern sometimes shows all over the parents, not
only in what they say but in the way they look and act. Typical of
the kind of advice that may be given to parents in either written or
oral form is the following:

> If your child bubbles along with frequent sputtering, hesitations,
> and repetitions of words, and, if he doesn't try to struggle or force
> his words out, there is little cause for alarm, especially if the child
> himself doesn't seem to show much concern about the way he
> talks. Help him to keep from learning to be alarmed about his
> way of talking.
>
> When your child sputters, it is easy and even natural for you
> to be concerned. But, it is difficult to keep from showing your con-
> cern. Try not to hold your breath. Try not to look anxious. The
> held breath or uplifted eyebrow should be replaced by a seemingly
> unconcerned, calm, patient attitude on your part. Let him know
> you are listening, but show concern for *what* he is saying—not for
> *how* he is saying it.

Parents should be instructed to refrain from any labeling of the
child's problem as stuttering or as a speech disorder. Although the
reasons for doing this should already be clear, the therapist should
make certain that the parent and teacher thoroughly understand
the rationale underlying this point. The parents should also be
helped to see the value of refraining from such activities as telling
the child to stop and start over, to slow down, or to use devices
for hiding or minimizing the stuttering. Additional parental suggestions may be phrased in this manner.

If he is told to stop his stuttering, or to think of what he is trying to say, or to take a deep breath, or given countless other warnings—all of which amount to "stop stuttering"—he will make a valiant effort to smooth out his speech and to keep the words coming out one after the other. In his effort to please you, he may begin to struggle on unfamiliar words or the will-o'-the-wisps of "proper grammar." After this happens a few times he may try to hide his embarrassment by talking less and less. Some children refuse to talk at all.

In an effort to help, well-meaning friends will sometimes suggest devices to promote fluent speech. These devices or tricks include snapping or tapping fingers, licking lips, blinking eyes, taking a breath, tapping a toe, or other contortions to start or finish a troublesome word. These tricks and devices never should be taught to a child. These mannerisms may help briefly, but in a short time, the child finds that their effectiveness wears off. Too often, when the tricks no longer help, they are not dropped but remain an habitual part of talking. Depending on the tricks he was taught, the child eventually will develop a bizarre pattern of blinking his eyes, snapping his fingers, or protruding his tongue when he is blocked —more grotesque than if he had simply forced his way through the word.

A mimeographed list of common do's and don'ts may be provided. The one that follows could serve as a pattern:

1. Don't let your child know you are worried about his way of talking.
2. Refrain from calling your child a stutterer or a stammerer; think of him as a normal child who presently appears to have some difficulty talking.
3. Look at your child when he talks and show by your expression that you are interested in what he has to say and that you enjoy talking with him.
4. Avoid practices that will put undue pressure on your child for good speech.
5. Be a good model for him to imitate in that you keep your own speech unhurried.
6. Refrain from teaching tricks or devices which you feel may help to reduce or eliminate his difficulty.
7. Don't try to persuade him to speak or recite before strangers or visitors. Let him do so if he wishes, but only then.
8. Don't ask him questions that require long answers. Word your questions so that definite short answers are possible.
9. If your child mentions frustration concerning his inability to talk fluently, reassure him that everyone finds it difficult to talk at times.

One of the best ways to satisfy the parents' need for "something to do" and at the same time to help them gain valuable insights into their child's problem is to supply them with observation checklists. Checklists make it easier for the parent to focus on particular aspects of the child's speech. By presenting parents with only one checklist at a time, it is possible to guide them in the types of observations you think most profitable at the time. When the parent returns with the completed list, a basis is formed for the beginning of constructive discussion.

Checklist A provides an opportunity for parents, who are openly critical of their child's effort to talk, to become aware of how often they engage in certain types of detrimental verbalizations.

### Checklist A

Arrange and carefully scrutinize your comments during a certain period each day.

Check each time you ask your child to
"Slow down!" _____
"Think of what you are going to say!" _____
"Take a deep breath!" _____
"Take it easy!" _____
"Don't try to say it all at once!" _____
Others _____
Check each time you talk about his stuttering
In front of him _____
To your spouse _____
To a friend or relative _____
Check each time you call his way of talking stuttering or stammering
In front of him _____
To your spouse _____
To a friend or relative _____

Sometimes parents need to know whether they talk in one certain way to their child more often than in another. In some cases we have known, this checklist has helped parents become acutely aware that most segments of their conversations fell in the undesirable "reprimanding, correcting" category: "Don't do this! Don't do that! Don't slouch! Keep your feet off the furniture! Don't you forget to be home on time! How many times do I have to tell you to turn lights out behind you?!"

The checklist system of directing observations is especially valuable in that it allows parents to notice their own shortcomings themselves without the therapist pointing them out.

CHECKLIST B

List below your comments to your child during a specific time of day, for example, just before he leaves for school tomorrow morning, during supper Wednesday, etc. Put a check mark down each time you use a particular type of comment. For example, if you say, "No, you can't stay up to watch TV," put a check mark under Denying Requests, etc.

| Date | Reprimanding, correcting | Approving, praising | Having fun with him | Denying requests |
|------|--------------------------|---------------------|---------------------|------------------|
|      |                          |                     |                     |                  |

The checklist shown in Figure C, a modification of the well known sociogram, is valuable for helping the parent to make observations of one of the common counterpressures to fluent speech—interruptions. Naturally, this form cannot be filled in with complete accuracy. The therapist may suggest that the parent study the form carefully before the time of the observation, then seek to fill it in in rough fashion immediately after the period of observation. In one family, the use of this checklist awakened the parents to the fact that the stuttering child was being continually interrupted by his siblings. In subsequent discussion, a policy of "speech manners" was established which greatly relieved the stuttering child of this source of frustration.

CHECKLIST C

Show by arrows the verbal exchanges occurring (*at lunch time*). Each time your child is interrupted while speaking, draw a short line across the arrow. ———|———▶

Each time he has to repeat his statement because of lack of attention on the part of the listener, make the arrow wavy. ∿∿∿▶

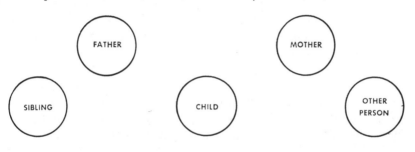

Checklist D enables the parent to observe more closely the relationship of the child's stuttering to possible sources of conflict. One father became aware of his part in his child's speech problem when he observed the frequent instances of stuttering in the child's conversations with him. This revelation led to a series of discussions with the father in which he found that he had not saved enough reserve strength and forbearance to greet and listen to his children when he got home at night. Eating a candy bar on the way home helped him to be less impatient about his supper. Awareness that his son looked forward to talking to him when he got home helped him to keep his nose out of his paper for at least fifteen minutes after he got home.

### CHECKLIST D

Check below each time your child does one of the following. If he stutters while performing one of these activities, place a star in the space.

| Asks permission | Relates an incident | Complains | Talks to father | Talks to mother |
|---|---|---|---|---|
| | | | | |

Checklist E serves to help parents select those factors which seem to be of greatest importance in modifying the increase in disfluency in the child's speech. This type of form leads easily into agreement on suitable measures to be undertaken in the home.

### CHECKLIST E

You have been keeping check-sheets on the verbal activity of your child. Now sit down as husband and wife and summarize the results of your observations and attempt to explain the instances where his stuttering seems to be increased. You can't be certain, so go ahead and guess.

The forms presented here are merely examples of the types of observational guides which the therapist can devise. As the parent gains more understanding of his role as it relates to the child's problem, various other kinds of checklists can be constructed. Their purpose is to direct the parent's observations to factors which might be pertinent, or which allow the parent to reach certain conclusions without the therapist having to point them out. These observational guides provide excellent starting places for profitable discussion.

Van Riper, in a book entitled *Your Child's Speech Problem,* includes a letter written by the mother of a child who had begun to stutter seriously. The letter is reproduced here because, as Van Riper points out, the letter summarizes the important things which parents of a beginning stutterer should do at home.

Dear Sir: You asked me to put down in a letter some of the things I told you we had done, and are still doing at home to help Bill overcome his stuttering. As I said, he now seems to have stopped it completely. Oh, once in awhile he hesitates but no more than I do. You know how you hesitate when you aren't sure of what you're going to say but nothing unusual. I mean he talks fine and straight now just like anybody else. I've been waiting for another siege of it to come but it's been over three months now since any showed up so I really think it's gone. You asked me to tell you about our family talks after Bill went to bed. Well, they had to do with some of the things you mentioned when you told me that afternoon that your waiting list was so long and you couldn't promise us an appointment for a long time. I just couldn't bear to wait the way Billy was stuttering so I sat my husband down every night and we took a look at ourselves. It was kind of hard at first but it got interesting after we broke the ice. Every night we would ask ourselves ten questions. Here they are:

1. Are we irritated or sore at each other or with Billy, How and why?

2. Are we talking too complicated, too much, too fast or too long so he thinks he has to talk like that too?

3. Are we putting the pressure on him to talk, asking him too many questions, wanting him to tell us too much: Lord, we were always doing this, we found. Over and over again in spite of good intentions.

4. Were we breaking up his speech by interrupting, nodding our heads before he's finished, not paying attention, leaving him to do something else while he was talking? There was plenty of this that we had to stop.

5. Were we making sure he knew we loved him, that he was awfully important to us? I guess we hadn't done enough along this line.

6. Had we been criticizing him too much, punishing him too much or making him feel he wasn't good enough? Every day we found some of this at first.

7. Did we let him blow off steam enough, get mad, or even be a baby? We found we'd been bottling up that poor kid more than we knew.

8. Had we cut out the excitement or anyway cut it down? We discovered that unplugging the TV helped and there were plenty of other ways to get a calmer house.

9. Had we been expecting too much of the kid? We had, every day, almost every hour.

10. Could the boy see that we were upset when he stuttered? This was the hardest of all to change but we changed it.

These were the questions we asked ourselves every night and I think this was the most important thing we did. Oh, I guess we also began to talk more slowly and quietly ourselves. I know I didn't talk as much or as fast and that was hard to change too. And we started listening, like you told us, to his good speech. At first there wasn't too much of it but it kept growing and soon that's all there was. Funny thing, too, we're all a lot calmer and happier. Anyway he's stopped so you can take his name off your waiting list (12:110-111).

### Providing Advice about Problems of Child Care Which Are Not Directly Speech Centered

So long as the therapist is providing information strictly about speech, he is on relatively safe ground; the parents and teacher usually recognize his competency in this area and expect him to guide and direct. But the environmental manipulations necessary for reducing the total problem of stuttering usually cannot be confined to suggestions for reacting to the stuttering itself. As was apparent in the checklists above, the conditions which may increase the child's tensions are often not speech centered. And even though the therapist must deal with non-speech-centered factors in the home, he must exercise caution when doing so. He must recognize that he is now on the borderline so far as his professional competency goes. For example, in some homes there may be a marital problem of sufficient tension to increase the child's tendency to stutter. The average speech therapist is probably not trained professionally to deal with problems of marital adjustment. Yet in particular instances, this kind of problem may be one of the most significant factors affecting the child's speech. How then should the speech therapist handle such problems which are not obviously speech centered and which tend to extend beyond his area of competence?

Beasley (1) has made the suggestion that the speech therapist use a form of "nondirective" counseling when dealing with parents of stutterers. The therapist, according to this article, should rephrase the parent's questions into another question back to the parent.

When dealing with non-speech-centered problems, this approach is often appropriate. Certainly, a nondirective approach is less likely to lead the therapist into dangerous waters.

In our opinion, the speech therapist has the responsibility of seeking to convince the parents of their need for referral to another profession when a problem is known or suspected, of making the proper referral, of providing the agency with the pertinent information which led to the referral, of informing the agency of how this problem is thought to affect the child's speech, of indicating any treatment procedures which are pertinent to the referral problem, and of arranging for the reception or transmission of information concerning the referral agency's diagnosis and treatment.

It is not always easy to convince parents that they should seek help from other agencies unless the parents talk about the problem to the speech therapist. In fact, unless the parent tells the therapist quite a bit, he may not know to whom the problem should be referred, or even if it is serious enough to demand referral. So, even though the speech therapist should not try to solve problems outside of his field, he must still investigate the existence of such problems and be aware of many things which do not directly affect the way the parents handle the child's speech. There are probably many different reasons for a child to be tense while speaking. It is the speech therapist's task to be on the lookout for these reasons and to do something about those that are found or suspected to exist. But "to do something" does not have to mean that we treat all such conditions. Unfortunately, speech therapists are easily tempted to play "psychologist" or "counselor" in all areas. This is especially true when the therapist has experienced success in counseling on speech centered problems. But there is danger in overplaying the role. The therapist without adequate preparation in psychology or counseling should not attempt to handle complex emotional problems. But, again, parents need to be encouraged to talk enough so that such problems can be recognized and appropriate referrals can be made.

Once a parent has related enough information to indicate that a serious non-speech-centered problem is obvious—the time is ripe for a referral. Perhaps this comes when the parent asks, "But what can I do about it?" Because this moment may not come again soon, the speech therapist might answer, "Well, I know some other folks with a similar problem who went to see Dr. Jones, our psychologist. He was able to help them. Would you like me to call Dr. Jones and see if I can make an appointment for you?" This act, performed matter-of-factly, may provide the incentive to begin working on a basic problem which has festered for some time.

Not all problems need to be referred. Often parents simply need reassurance that they are doing a good job, or a little more understanding of why they react to their child's stuttering as they do. In such instances, it is appropriate for the speech therapist to utilize basic mental hygiene suggestions and concepts.

### Counseling Procedures

There is considerable merit in following a general pattern for counseling sessions with parents. Sander points out that the child should be examined before the counseling sessions. "It would seem both futile and unrealistic, for example, to attempt to convince a parent that her child's nonfluencies are perfectly natural if he is already reacting to his speech, struggling, or displaying an habitually excessive degree of tension." (8:264). Brown (3) recommends that the child should be examined in the presence of his parents and then again without them present. When the therapist first sees a child in school, the examination, of course, comes first.

. Arrangements for parent interviews, the place, and number of visits depend on so many circumstances that no attempt to elaborate will be made here except to stress that they are of absolute necessity if the speech of the child is to be modified. Also, what is said here may also apply to the teacher. Furthermore, the therapist can never assume that when the parents are concerned about the child's speech his teacher will be too, and vice versa. The therapist must check this carefully.

Schuell outlines the pattern for a series of interviews thus:

> *The First Interview:* The object of the first interview is necessarily to gain as much information as possible about the parents as well as about the child. The parents must not be placed on the defensive and must be encouraged to talk as freely as possible.
> *The Second Interview:* In the second interview it is usually possible to find out the ideas which the parents have held about stuttering, to answer some of their questions about it, and to begin to give them information about the way stuttering begins and develops. It is also necessary to give them something constructive which they can begin to do.

*The. Third Interview:* In this interview the speech correctionist is able to go over with the parents the data gathered by assignments, and from them and the parents' comments, form an idea of what is to be worked on or changed (9).

Perhaps the therapist would be wise to utilize Johnson's suggestion—begin as the physician does—with the parent's complaint. Although the following illustration pertains to a patient coming with his own problems, it appears applicable to parents or teachers who come for help for a child's speech.

It is usually true that when a person first comes to a clinic . . . he wants, above everything else, to get something off his chest. He wants to talk: He may not be ready to "Tell all," he may not know quite how to say what he has to say, but at least he does not come just to read the magazine on the waiting room table. No unnecessary obstacles should be put in his way. He should not be stopped by a receptionist who is clearly more interested in the clinic's filing system than she is in his anxieties. Certainly no clinician who has ever been a case himself would begin by putting the distraught individual through the cold inquisition of a standardized case history interview, or by giving him a test (6:393).

An atmosphere should be created in which it is easy for parents to tell about the child's problem. This may be done by displaying. interest and understanding, by indicating through questions that the therapist wants to hear more—more about the child and his problems, and more about why the parents are concerned and what they have done to help. An "I see" answer should be used only if it tends to elicit more information. During the first interview, it is better to stay on the side of "tell me more about what you mean when you say . . ." or "I'm not quite sure I understand."

But, during the first counseling session, the therapist should be more than just an interested listener. The parents expect reassurance. Such reassurance does not usually come from quick statements to the effect that "your child will be all right." The reassurance comes from their knowing they have brought their child to the proper person—to an individual who understands this kind of condition and who will, at the very least, know *something* that can be done about it.

Before the first session is completed, the parents should be informed of the diagnosis (even though it may be tentative) and be provided with some indication of the treatment to be followed. As a rule, any prolonged discussion of the nature of stuttering or the nature of speech and language development should be postponed for later conferences. There is one exception to this. Because of the tremendous. importance of the parents' reactions to the child's stuttering, it may be helpful to give parents some "do's" and "don'ts" at the first session, even though more detailed explanations and discussions may be reserved for further conferences.

In most instances, the information brought out by the parent during the first conference will concern the speech problem directly. Although the therapist may detect possible tensions in the home which affect the child's speech, it is usually wise to postpone exploration of these conditions until later. There is a good reason for this. In most instances, the parents initially view their child's problem entirely as a *speech* problem. Darley (4) found that only 16 per cent of the parents studied said that they considered the role of parents to be of causal importance in the development of stuttering. Parents are not always ready to see the child's stuttering as a problem to which they are directly related. To approach the parents at this stage with questions or suggestions which imply the necessity for basic changes in the way they behave toward their child or each other will often lead to resistance. Parents are likely to be more receptive later, after relationships have been established more firmly and after the basic nature of stuttering and speech and language development have been discussed.

The therapist should also be aware of probable differences in parents' receptivity depending on (a) whether or not the child has previously been examined elsewhere; (b) whether the parents seek services of the therapist or come to the conference at the request of the therapist; and (c) the type of "image" which the therapist has built up in the eyes of the community.

### Direct Versus Environmental Therapy Approaches

Since the distinction between primary and secondary stuttering was first made by Bluemel (2), it has been traditional to recommend indirect or environmental therapy (working only through parents and teachers) for the primary stutterer, and direct therapy (face-to-face contacts of the child with the therapist—reference being made to the speech symptoms) for the secondary stutterer. As stated by Eisenson and Ogilvie, "The primary stutterer should be given no direct speech therapy or any other form of therapy that he can relate to his speech. Nothing should be done or said to the child that suggests that his speech is in any way in need of change " (5:217).In discussing secondary stuttering in the same text Eisenson and Ogilvie state, "The secondary stutterer . . . is aware that his speech is atypical, and has reactions to himself and to his environment in terms of his awareness and evaluation of his speech. Therapeutic objectives, therefore, include a modification of the speech pattern as well as modification of the attitudes that the stutterer has developed toward himself, his speech, and his environment " (5:224).

This dichotomy of therapy approaches presents problems, however. As pointed out in Chapter Two, it is extremely difficult and perhaps inaccurate to classify all stutterers into two groups, primary and secondary. Furthermore, it is inappropriate to have only two types of therapy for all stutterers (3:51). There are many different levels and degrees of directness. A therapist may work with a child in a face-to-face, regularly scheduled session and never mention the word stuttering to the child. With another the therapist may find it to the child's advantage to speak of stuttering but restrict himself solely to discussions about "how everyone stutters," etc. A therapist may work with still another child and concentrate heavily upon modifying the secondary aspects of his stuttering, e.g., decreasing fears of specific words, or even analyzing the child's basic needs to stutter.

A similar problem of classification is encountered when we discuss indirect therapy with primary stutterers. If by working indirectly, one means working with the important persons in an individual's environment, then most therapists would agree that such an approach is useful for most secondary stutterers as well as for those classified as primary. Also, because some children who are just beginning to stutter misarticulate certain speech sounds, it is often imperative that they receive speech help. Thus, the therapist works directly with the child's speech, even though he does not treat his "stuttering." Some beginning stutterers who are unaware that they speak improperly can profit from direct attempts to facilitate fluency.

The question of whether to employ direct or indirect therapy with the stutterer is probably ill-phrased. Perhaps it would be more appropriate to ask, "How directive should the therapy program for this child be at this time?" In other words, the question of direct versus environmental is a matter of degree, not a simple either-or question.

Some of the major levels of "directness" in therapy are enumerated below. The therapy approaches increase in the degree of directness reading down the list.

1. *No direct involvement with the child.* All therapy is done through persons such as the child's parents and teachers. Generally, the parents and teachers are instructed to do their utmost to see that the child is kept unaware of any feelings that his speech is different.
2. *Direct contact between child and therapist but with no attention being focused on speech production.* At this level, children may be enrolled in "play groups" wherein the primary purpose is to observe the child. Children may also be engaged in creative dramatics activities with other children. *Desensitization Therapy\** may be thought of as fitting into this category, for the purpose of the activities are unknown to the child. So far as the child is concerned, he is playing games, not improving speech production.
3. *Direct contact with attention focused on speech improvement but not directly on stuttering.* This level is a little more directive than the previous one since the child will be aware that he is in speech therapy seeking to improve his speech. No mention need be made of stuttering, and the child need not know that fluency is a therapy goal, even though the activities are planned with that goal in mind. Examples of speech centered activities which fit into this category are fluency-enhancing approaches such as choral reading, rhythmic speaking, and talking-and-writing activities.
4. *Direct therapy with the child's attention focused on reducing stuttering but with labeling and complexity of techniques held to a minimum.* In instances where the child is highly aware of his stuttering, but where he has not developed a highly complex symptomatology, the therapy of choice is often supportive in nature. The therapist acknowledges to the child that he recognizes his stutterings. Little emphasis is placed upon the emotional content of the term *stuttering* and control techniques are kept at a minimum. The child is encouraged to stutter easily—to go ahead and let stuttered words come out but without "pushing at them quite so hard." At this level, however, strong attempts to encourage the child to "admit to others that he stutters" or detailed techniques of control such as learning loose contacts, pull-outs, or cancellations would not be utilized. The therapist may use some of these approaches but can work them into therapy without calling undue attention to them. Justification would be based on the child's need for a basic attitude toward his way of talking and some

---

\* Desensitization therapy, as described by Van Riper, refers to a set of procedures designed to increase a child's ability to withstand pressures which interfere with fluent speech (11:371-73).

help in handling troublesome words in order to eliminate or minimize some of the behaviors which bring him social penalties. The therapist by indirection attempts to avoid stigmatizing the child with a self-concept of "being a stutterer."

5. *Direct therapy with emphasis upon stuttering and with considerable attention being directed at the attitudes connected with stuttering and at the maladaptive speech behaviors associated with the stuttering.* At this level the stutterer is encouraged to bring his stuttering out into the open—to stutter on purpose. His difficult words are analyzed and different ways of approaching them are suggested. As a rule, this degree of directness is reserved for the chronic stutterer—for the child whose self-concept already is that of "being a stutterer" and whose stuttering behavior is involved and well-learned.

It is apparent that each of these levels of directness contains many sublevels. Some of the factors which affect the therapist's decision as to choice of levels are discussed below.

### Factors in Making Decisions as to the Relative Degree of Directive Therapy Approaches to Use

Although a decision on *how* directive to be is much more difficult to make than whether or not to be directive, there are certain guide lines which can be employed to aid in these decisions. It is not a matter of pure guesswork, but of balancing several factors in order to arrive at a decision. In the first place, the age of the child will help in the decision. In general, the younger the child, the better it is to concentrate on environmental approaches and to be less directive. The younger the child, the more likely it is that he will "forget" unfavorable speech experiences. With most preschool stutterers, therapy is limited to environmental manipulations irrespective of the severity of the stuttering pattern or the child's apparent degree of awareness. With children in the primary grades, we are inclined to rely very strongly on low-level indirect therapy procedures even though the child may display secondary stuttering patterns.

Another factor influencing the degree of directness is the amount and severity of forcing and avoidance patterns observed in the child. The more often such patterns occur, the more direct therapy should be.

The child's awareness of his stuttering is an important factor. The more aware the child is of his stuttering, the more feasible it is to use a direct approach. But, simply because a child displays some recognition of his speaking difficulty, it is not enough to conclude that a direct approach is the only answer. The authors have seen their own children (who are not stutterers nor could they be classified as stutterers) express annoyance and frustration over developmental disfluencies which interfered with their ability to communicate easily and readily. Upon asking children why they were brought in to see us in our respective speech clinics, we have heard several dozen say, "I'm here because I stutter." These same children display otherwise complete ignorance about what was meant by the word *stuttering*. But, we have also seen a number of children who did not associate their way of talking with stuttering, who habitually employed avoidance devices, thus belying the fact that they were unaware. In spite of this, in general we reserve advanced direct therapy approaches for the child who is obviously convinced that he is "a stutterer."

Sometimes therapy planning is influenced by one or both parents being unable to carry out the requirements of therapy. Perhaps home conditions are such that there is no reasonable chance to remove disturbing influences. Perhaps the child's grandmother keeps insisting that the boy doesn't need to talk like that around her. Perhaps the instability of a parent may not respond to psychiatric treatment, Alcoholics Anonymous, or the threat of the juvenile courts—depending on the nature of the instability. Some parents are too deeply involved in other problems: unemployment, separation, recent death, or illness. Some parents are unimaginative, some are too rigid, some too anxious. In these instances, when the parents want their child helped, and when for some sound reason it appears unwise to leave the treatment up to the child's parents, direct therapy at a slightly higher level than would ordinarily be employed is indicated. Prognosis will be poor, for the therapist is working against considerable odds.

As a rule, then, it is better to begin therapy at the lowest approach level which holds promise of altering the child's speech and stuttering reactions. Therapy can always be made more directive if a particular indirect approach is unsuccessful, but reducing the amount of directness will not always be possible, since increased awareness and confrontation with stutterings occur as the level of directness is stepped up.

## References

1. BEASLEY, J. "Relationship of Parental Attitudes to Development of Speech Problems," *Journal of Speech and Hearing Disorders*, XXI (1956), 317-21.
2. BLUEMEL, C. S. "Primary and Secondary Stammering," *Quarterly Journal of Speech*, XVIII (1932), 187-200.
3. BROWN, S. F. "Advising Parents of Early Stutterers," *Pediatrics* (1949), 170-75.
4. DARLEY, F. L. "The Relationship of Parental Attitudes and Adjustments to the Development of Stuttering," In *Stuttering in Children and Adults*, W. Johnson and R.R. Leutenegger (eds.), (Minneapolis: University of Minnesota Press, 1955).
5. EISENSON, J., and M. OGILVIE. *Speech Correction in the Schools* (New York: The Macmillan Company, 1957).
6. JOHNSON, W. *People in Quandaries* (New York: Harper & Row, Publishers, 1946).
7. POOLE, I. "Genetic Development of Articulation of Consonant Sounds in Speech," *Elementary English Review*, XI (1934), 159-61.
8. SANDER, E. K. "Counseling Parents of Stuttering Children," *Journal of Speech and Hearing Disorders*, XXIV (1959), 262-71.
9. SCHUELL, H. "Working with Parents of Stuttering Children," *Journal of Speech and Hearing Disorders*, XIV (1949), 251-54.
10. *Stuttering: Its Prevention*. (Memphis, Tenn.: Speech Foundation of America, 1962).
11. VAN RIPER, C. *Speech Correction: Principles and Methods*, Fourth Ed. (Englewood Cliffs, N.J.: Prentice-Hall, Inc., 1963).
12. ———. *Your Child's Speech Problems* (New York: Harper & Row, Publishers, 1961).

*Chapter Four*

## The Modification of Transitional
## Stuttering (Phase Two)

*In this phase of the disorder, the child's difficulty is essentially chronic even though it may fluctuate in severity and may even disappear briefly from time to time. This transitional stage of development usually occurs when the child is around six or seven years of age. Although for some individuals there may be a tendency to have more difficulty in certain situations, the child stutters primarily when he "talks fast" and "gets excited." The moments of stuttering now have attached themselves to the major parts of speech. Although the child calls himself a stutterer, he speaks freely and shows little concern about his stuttering. Therapy for children at this stage may be environmental or may involve face-to-face contacts between the therapist and the child. Face-to-face techniques will vary some in how "direct" they are but in general will be relatively nondirective.*

At the transitional stage of stuttering development, it is still well within reason to aim at freeing the child's speech of disfluency and freeing his mind from the necessity of viewing his way of talking as stuttering. A minimal goal is to prevent, insofar as possible, the growth and development of visible and audible symptoms of stuttering and to insure an attitudinal climate that will minimize chances that the child might eventually view his speech as a handicap.

The objectives also include the following considerations:

> The child's parents and teachers need help to understand the approach to be followed in therapy. Since therapy may or may not be indirect, the child may or may not be included in discussions of therapy planning.
> The child's sense of worth and general well-being need to be fortified and enhanced.
> Ample and successful opportunities for talking must be provided. An effort must be made to build the child's confidence in being able to talk well.

### Planning for Systematic Therapy

Even though the child whose speech is diagnosed as Phase Two stuttering calls his way of talking "stuttering," he usually shows little or no concern about the way he talks. One basic requisite of therapy is to insure that his self-concept does not change unfavorably as a result of growing concern about his way of talking. Because the level of concern is low for many children at this developmental phase, special consideration should be given as to which children should receive systematic speech therapy outside of the routine of the regular classroom. The kind of therapy that should be provided him at this stage, in or out of the speech therapy session, will of necessity be supportive in nature, i.e., it will consist mainly of providing the child with ways of doing things successfully. Not all of the emphasis will necessarily be on talking. Depending on the child, emphasis in therapy may be on increasing self-confidence or perfecting learning skills. With some it may also be necessary to emphasize the relearning or modifica-

69

tion of maladaptive behavior involving speech. Planning for therapy should allow an opportunity for the child's teacher and parents to discuss the pros and cons concerning the features of the management program. The clinician should take into consideration whether the child's parents are for or against, resistant or cooperative, understanding or unimaginative, concerning the possible advantages and disadvantages of taking him out of his classroom for speech help. If the decision is reached that the child will not be taken from his classroom for speech help, the therapist, in cooperation with the child's parents and teacher, should plan a program which will not only minimize the possibility of an increase in stuttering symptoms but also provide a program of speech improvement that may be beneficial not only to the child who stutters, but also to the other children in the classroom.

At this stage of development, it is better to stay on the safe side, that is, not take the child out of his room for speech therapy if there is doubt about the wisdom of doing so. Several examples will help in determining by which criteria this decision should be made. The child who calls himself a stutterer, but whose speech symptoms are not severe and whose general adjustment to his teacher and classmates is good, may profit by therapy outside of his regular class, but there still remains a danger of establishing doubts in his mind about his ability to talk well. Therefore, this child is probably a doubtful candidate for therapy outside his classroom. Doubtful cases are also at the other extreme—for example, a child whose general classroom adjustment is poor and whose poor potential for adjustment may not permit him to relate to a speech therapist (or to other children if group speech therapy is under consideration). Certainly, no Phase Two stutterer should be placed with Phase Four stutterers in a speech therapy group, and only in the more severe stages of development should he be placed with Phase Three stutterers.

However, a Phase Two stutterer should not be considered a doubtful case for speech therapy simply because he has not developed such advanced features of stuttering as word substitutions and word and situation fears. Some clinicians avoid placing these children in special classes because of their fear that a more severe form of stuttering may appear. Bloodstein (1) points out that the fact that a child's difficulty has become chronic makes it fair to presume that he is now in urgent need of some kind of systematic therapy, and the fact that he already considers himself a stutterer makes it unlikely that any harm will come to him from the discovery that someone else also regards him as one.

Thus, therapy at this level may be environmental, that is, conducted through the child's parents and teachers without involving the child, or it may involve direct contact between the child and speech therapist. If child centered, the focus of attention at this developmental stage may or may not involve specifics of speech production. If it does, the child's attention is not drawn directly to his stuttering.

### Parent Counseling

Whether the child is entered into direct therapy or not, a program of parent counseling should be carried out whenever possible along the lines suggested for Phase One stuttering—with one important difference. In the modification of incipient stuttering, one avoids using the label "stuttering." In Phase Two, the child admits to his stuttering and uses the word "stuttering" to refer to his way of talking. While there is considerable merit in making a concentrated effort to refrain from applying this label of "stuttering" to early stages of behavior, someone, somewhere along the line, and possibly the child himself, will note that society has a ready-made name for the behavior—and use it. When this happens care should be taken to point out that what he calls stuttering may not turn out to be stuttering after all. At this point the word does not mean to the child what it means to an adult. But, it is important that additional negative semantic valence not be added to the meaning of the word through vigorous denial that the label is improper. If the child calls what he does "stuttering," calm acquiescence and an attitude of unconcerned acceptance will do much to put the behavior in a proper perspective. Acceptance of the fact, without protest, may be the important first step in an open-minded orientation to the fact that some kinds of stuttering are not like other kinds of stuttering. This is not to say that the child should not be encouraged to discard the label at a later time, but it does mean that due respect should be shown for the child's perceptiveness of what he is doing and his sensitivity to what society calls the thing he is doing—rightly or wrongly.

Careful observation of the manner in which a child uses the label "stuttering" is a good indicator of the importance he attaches to it or wants to attach to it. Certainly if he refers to his speech casually and without outward concern, no one else should refrain from using the term simply because it has negative connotations. A child at this stage of development will not be as concerned about using the word as are his parents, or even his speech clinician, because he does not know nor does he need to be taught about later stages.*

If the child is refreshingly naïve about his speech condition, the speech clinician, the teacher, and the child's parents should not be concerned about doing possible damage to him. But, parents must have the courage of their convictions. Appreciation, acceptance, and affection for an individual and his individuality constitute the soil in which security grows. Additional tolerance must be added whenever any of these ingredients is missing or in short supply.

Although the most common complaint leveled against parents is that they show too much concern when their child shows signs of stuttering, some few parents create a different kind of problem when they do not eventually admit their concern to their child. Some children advance to the stage where they splutter and struggle in obvious distress while their parents stand by without any outward sign of awareness, much less concern. Usually these parents are successfully hiding their very real and deep-seated concern in a conscientious effort to prevent the further development of stuttering symptoms. In Chapter Three, a wait-and-watch approach was strongly advocated. There are, however, detrimental forces at work on a child that sometimes cannot be foreseen or controlled. Sometimes the symptoms persist or even grow in frequency of occurrence in spite of inspired cooperative efforts on the part of the parents and teachers. One of the dangers in this wait-and-watch approach is that parents do not always know when

---

* Avoidance of excessive use of the term "stuttering" still is of continued value whenever possible and these comments are consistent with the comments concerning the inadvisability of diagnosing or labeling the behavior as stuttering when first noticed. Note that the label sticks and the behavior worsens when both the word "stuttering" and the behavior it refers to are considered undesirable. Words which tend to describe what he does when he repeats words or finds his lips pressed together are the words that really say more about his present condition, and these words are always the preferred ones. Tangible acts such as these are easier to combat than intangibles covered by abstract words like "stuttering" which often imply that a more pervasive condition exists.

and how to shift from a show of unconcern to helpful awareness.
Usually the shift should be made when the symptoms do not abate after a reasonable effort has been made to modify them indirectly. If the stutterings increase in severity or frequency, and especially, if, along with the increase, the child has stated that he stutters or begins to show increased signs of embarrassment or confusion, the air should be cleared.

Sometimes parents resist confrontation with the idea that the child really is stuttering. During parent counseling, it should be pointed out that the child carries an unreasonably heavy burden when his parents do not acknowledge that he is doing something unusual. It should be pointed out that their child may even progress more quickly through the developmental stages of stuttering if he gets the impression that he must battle alone against the strange thing that he thinks is happening to him when he talks. He may even come to conclude that he can never truly win or even deserve his parents' love unless he rids himself of his impediment. He may think along these lines:

> I know that I am having one awful time talking, but strangely enough no one else appears to think so. I hate this thing I'm doing, but no one else seems to care, maybe everyone else has given up on me. Maybe what I do is so bad no one dares mention it.

Parents should be able to talk about what their child is doing without feeling that his speech will get worse because they give it a name. They should be able to give the child the hope he so badly needs by saying, "Yes, you are having some trouble talking now, but you won't always talk like this. We all have difficulty talking at times—we all get our tongues tangled up at times. The important thing is not to become tense about it when we do get tangled up." A difference should be admitted without subterfuge or double talk, because by now he realizes he doesn't talk the way others talk. The ability to think and talk unemotionally about what the child is doing ties in with the next few remarks about fluency and disfluency.

*Fluency Versus Disfluency*

When the parents of a child who stutters are asked what results they expect from therapy, they invariably state the obvious; what they want and expect is fluency, in other words, no stuttering.

The same predictable answer is also obtained when the same question is asked of an older child or young adult who stutters. Thus, by definition, stuttering and disfluency become the opposites of fluency and nonstuttering. When this criterion is applied in a judgment of whether therapy is successful, therapy is judged to be successful only when there is a presence of fluency and an absence of stuttering.

The clinician must keep his eyes open to the obvious pitfall in this line of reasoning; that is, that the presence of any disfluency at any time may be pounced on as evidence that therapy has not been successful. The therapist must be careful to assure through his parent counseling sessions that he is not attempting therapy in an evaluational system that might possibly snap shut on him for this reason. Not that the clinician won't keep fluency in mind as a goal, but this goal can be more readily achieved when the presence of a varying amount of disfluency is tolerated for what it is—the normal consequences and by-products of using an incompletely learned avenue of communication in a verbally competitive society.

The clinician, as well as the child and his parents and teachers, should remember that freedom from fear is a more important goal than freedom from disfluency. A child can learn to adapt his speaking rate to his optimum fluency level much easier than he can dispel the fear that arises after stuttering has become an habitual manner of reacting.

*Disfluencies*

Disfluencies take several forms, and many disfluencies cannot and should not be equated with stuttering. It should be pointed out that society tolerates a certain amount of disfluency and actually expects it under certain circumstances. In most instances, pauses and retrials are the result of earnest efforts to remember an appropriate word, or the result of sorting among several words of similar meaning to find the word with the most suitable shade of meaning. Fumbles and new starts are necessary when undertaking complicated directions or explanations. "And uh"—"and er" are often the speaker's signal to his audience that his speaking motor is still running and for the moment he is trying to get his thought gears engaged. This latter behavior is especially prevalent when someone is under pressure to relinquish the floor or when he must compete for his audience's rarely undivided attention. If this then is disfluency, what is fluency?

*Fluency*

Fluency too is several things. Fluency is not just an absence of stuttering, nor is it simply the absence of disfluency. The following is an expression of the meaning of fluency that is much broader than "the opposite of nonfluency":

> Fluency is a smooth flow of words, aptly selected, which express an idea or sentiment economically or affluently, according to circumstances. Fluency is learned and develops and changes through experience. Fluency does not spring full grown into existence but falters at first just like a young bird learning to fly and stumbles just as does a young child learning to walk. Fluency isn't always appropriate for the expression of strong emotions such as surprise, shock, or dismay, nor is it always the bedfellow of sincerity. Fluency in its most grandiose form is sometimes called eloquence.

One can expect that the child's parents and his teachers have been exposed to the compelling dictum of advertisers to their potential customers, "Don't accept a substitute." The wise clinician can adopt the tactics of the advertisers to the extent that he expends every effort to spell out what the genuine products are, i.e., fluency and disfluency. This type of "hard sell" will warrant the necessary effort and will assure fewer relapses, a healthy climate in which speech can be experimented with and enjoyed, and above all, it will insure that his speech will be acceptable to the child and to his most important consumers. But, before more is said about this, some other considerations in therapy should be taken up.

### Therapy Specifics

A wait-and-watch approach for a child in the first stages of stuttering contains another inherent danger in that it is possible to wait too long. In addition to the problem of emotional overlay, a child may grow accustomed to talking in a pattern marked by hesitations and interruptions. This is to say that disfluent speech

can quickly become habitual for him just as fluent speech becomes habitual for another child.

When a child first begins to stutter, a wait-and-watch approach
is advisable. But, when the symptoms persist for several months in
spite of behind-the-scenes environmental manipulations, when the
symptoms increase in frequency, when they flare up when he talks
fast or gets excited, or when other signs appear that the stutterings
are on the increase rather than on the decline, then direct therapy
specifics are called for.

One way to view stuttering behavior is as a learned response to
a stimulus of "speech anxiety." Viewed in this manner, the problem becomes one of the learning theorists' $S-R$ bond or conditioned response. With this concept in mind, the child at this
stage would appear to be exhibiting behavior which, although
not yet conditioned to the "habit" stage (Hull's $sHr$), is certainly
occurring often enough to increase the habit potential. To paraphrase from Hull's theory of learning (2), the stimulus of anxiety
leads to a response of excess tension in the speech musculature.
Each time this particular pattern is repeated—the combination of
anxiety, tension, and subsequent anxiety reduction—the possibility
of excess tension becoming habitually attached to the stimulus of
anxiety is increased. The Phase Two stutterer may be thought of
as one who has repeated this particular pattern often enough for
it to approach—but not quite reach—habit strength. The point
here is that the frequent occurrence of stuttering behavior does
call for direct measures. The more frequently this type of response
is elicited, the greater the chance of this form of behavior becoming habitual.

Interestingly enough, children of the same age level as those who
are beginning to stutter, but who have articulation problems, work
actively in face-to-face therapy together with a speech therapist to
overcome their deviations. Curiously, when the question arises
about whether direct therapy will embarrass the child or make him
self-conscious, the question is most frequently asked by the parents
or teachers—not by the speech therapist. The speech therapist
in his justification claims the future welfare of the child is at
stake. He feels that the hazards of temporary unpleasantness, embarrassment, or self-consciousness are not as important as the possibility that the speech deviations may become habitual. The
matter of the child's ability to withstand the constant frustration

of "Huh? Say that again!" is taken into account. Cautions to the effect that a child may refuse to talk or become shy or withdrawn unless therapy is undertaken are standard statements in speech pathology textbooks. Only in the literature concerning stuttering is an appeal made to wait-and-watch. If a waiting-out period is mentioned, it is mentioned only to determine misarticulations which tend to disappear through maturation. When the discussion is concerned with school-age children, the discussion usually centers around the administrative problems concerned with reducing heavy caseloads.

Therapy specifics for articulation problems are legion. The therapist is able to point out and help eliminate an *S* or *R* error and does not feel that the child will be threatened by the collapse of his speaking ability. The therapist recognizes the need to get in and do the necessary job of correction and then to get out— to provide therapy only when needed and only until that time when the child can carry on his own self-correction. Also, the therapist quickly learns that correction rarely provides adverse embarrassment or extreme self-consciousness. Few children balk at speech therapy. Most children welcome the opportunity for constructive growth afforded by active participation in speech improvement sessions. When resistance is found, it is often because a child attaches little importance to the necessity for improvement, not because the corrective process reflects unfavorably on the child's self-image.

Some children start to stutter while undergoing articulation therapy. This is a calculated risk that a therapist and the child's parents must take. When stuttering occurs, it serves as a signal that conditions apparently operate in the child's background that need further investigation. It signals for a prompt review and possible revision of therapy procedures. It is not necessarily a signal to call off therapy. Unquestionably, means for shoring up his speaking ability are needed. The same indirect and environmental approaches which have been previously mentioned are appropriate for these children. But, other means are available to take the sting out of the stutterings. However, in order to do so, the stuttering will have to be touched.

Several succeeding chapters of this book are devoted to means for confrontation with the actual stuttering symptoms and for providing face-to-face therapy specifics.

## Providing a Program of General Speech Improvement

Today's schools are talking schools. To be able to profit fully from modern educational approaches it is more important than ever before that a child be willing and able to talk. Ample provisions are made for children to talk. Today's teachers are rarely concerned because a child whispers in class. Whispering, an offense against classroom decorum a decade or so ago, isn't anywhere near the crime it was in the little red schoolhouse because healthy outlets for pent-up speech are available to children in our modern schools. Instead, today's teachers are more apt to express concern over children who don't do much talking—children who may be referred to as nonparticipators.

School does little to dampen a modern child's enthusiasm for talking and does much to sharpen his desire, willingness, and ability to talk. School discipline still amounts to restricting the amount of spontaneous talking a child does, even as it did years ago. But, the approaches being followed today in school do not condone the repressive "speak only when spoken to" measures of yesteryear. A healthy respect for children as unique, talking individuals is shown in the emphasis placed on outlets for talking. Almost universally, modern school curricula include provision for "show and tell," discussion periods, cooperative planning, creative dramatics, and the like.

For many children the beginning of school serves as an introduction to an aspect of speech that hasn't been stressed before. Modern preschool children are encouraged to talk, so they talk from the time they get out of bed in the morning until they go to bed at night. Most parents will attest that their children find it difficult to turn off their talking switches—and with good reason. From infancy, a word incidentally that means "without speech," most children are encouraged to talk. A child's first coos and "da-da's" are joyously exclaimed over and the more they say the more enthusiastic are their listeners. Children's first words and expressions are eagerly anticipated and modern parents openly show their delight in the fact that their children talk. Only rarely are today's children "seen and not heard." (On the contrary— someone, undoubtedly a crank, has pointed out that children today are not only seen and heard, but heard, and heard, and heard.)

Today's teachers deliberately attempt to restructure the preschool system which operates to reward talking. Whereas our preschool children are encouraged to talk freely at home, school children are rewarded for *listening* as well as talking.*

School is the very first place some children find where they will be rewarded for not talking—for stopping talking. At home, the talking of preschool children is mostly "middle," without much beginning or end. They rarely start talking because they rarely stop talking. At school, for example, in "show and tell," they find that they are rewarded for standing up, starting to talk, saying something, and stopping. They are persuaded that it is important to find an end for their short speech so that someone else can have a turn at talking. Although a successful beginning may have started at home, children find that at school they are consistently rewarded for listening without interrupting while someone else talks. Stress is placed upon being not only good talkers but also good listeners, and they are rewarded for not only being good listeners to teacher but good listeners to their classmates as well. At school, too, they find that if they are to get an audience, what they say must be important enough to earn the ear of a critical audience—but it is an audience that is made up of listeners—listeners their own age who know how to reward the interesting talker with eager attention.

Thus, it may be seen that most children thrive and increase in their ability to speak well in today's schools, not only because of the favorable conditions for verbal expression found in modern schools, but because of the practice they get in the security of their homes as preschoolers. These children bring to school an ability to talk based on rewarded, unhampered, copious output. The light restrictions placed on their way of talking at school do little to inhibit them as talkers and are designed to permit growth in their talking skills as befits children in an age where the necessity to communicate has never before been so important.

Children who stutter, however, do not always come out of home

---

* After visiting schools in forty-two states, Wilt found that children were expected to listen to one thing or another 57.5 per cent of the school day. At the kindergarten-primary level the median amount of time presumably is well over 60 per cent because so many of the daily activities revolve around the spoken word. [Miriam E. Wilt, "A Study of teacher awareness of listening as a factor in elementary education," *Journal of Educational Research*, XLIII, 626-36 (April, 1950).]

backgrounds conducive to the growth and development of secure speech as has just been described. Mother and father may demand speech rather than encourage speech. They may tend to reward the child for perfection in speech rather than for quantity or adequacy. They may even require that speech be used as a precision tool that will enable him to perform a job of work rather than as a pleasant thing to do, something to be experimented with and enjoyed.

At any stage of stuttering, the child misses out on the rewards of feeling a free flow of words coming from his mouth when there are constraints causing him to wonder if he is going to be interrupted or corrected, or whether he will break down because he runs out of words to express his ideas.

Some children who stutter learn to talk late and are more or less insecure about talking because their speech is generally unintelligible. Many of them frequently encounter, "Huh?— What?— Say that again?" These children, some of them at least, quickly join the "It's Better to Remain Quiet and Thought Dumb than to Speak and Remove All Doubt Club." Some of them must compete unsuccessfully with brothers and sisters. These children may find it almost impossible to get a word in edgewise.

> I was the oldest of a family of six—three brothers and two sisters. We all did well in school. I remember someone once saying to my parents that every one of their children seemed to be brighter than the next one. Everybody talked well except me. It was bedlam around our house. Everyone talked at once and had a hilarious good time doing so. My first memory of having trouble talking was when I was trying to tell about something at the dinner table—I never have been able to remember what. I kept saying over and over, "Let me tell you something." When I finally did get a chance to talk all I could say was "I-I-I-I-I," because I had forgotten what it was I was trying to say.

An unfortunate aspect of our society is the premium we put on the quick retort, or snappy comeback, and the tendency to hold the answerer in higher regard than we do the asker of questions. Even with our enlightened approach to communication and education, we still find in our schools that there is a tendency to judge a person's scholarship, if not his intelligence, on the basis of the latency period between the time when the instructor points his finger at the end of the question and the time a student's mouth begins to make answering noises. The idea seems to be, "the shorter the silence, the higher the intelligence." The hesitant child is too often the loser if exposed to too much of this kind of pressure.

The verbal bandit is also a constant threat in our society. The interrupter who eagerly awaits the smallest opening to wedge in a correction or his own version of the so-called facts, or simply a chance to hold forth on his own, is a well known fixture in our society. And so again we find our way back to the availability of disfluency in our society.

Unless a person is well equipped to steal someone else's thunder, he may succumb to the pressure of verbal competition and generally lose out on the give-and-take of communication. It is small wonder that there are so many "and's" in connected speech. It is necessary to keep going until one runs out of breath in altogether too many conversations, especially when several people are trying to express their views at once. To start a new sentence may offer the verbal bandit the tiny opening he needs in which to interrupt and take over. In a verbally competitive household, some children literally never get a chance to finish a thought. People who fall into a passive role and don't take an active part in the give-and-take of everyday talking miss out on the legwork necessary to be able to think on their feet. Children learning to stutter aren't the only ones who miss out on this practice as illustrated by the comments of a twenty-two-year-old, nonstuttering male.

> For me, practice teaching was living hell. Why I ever thought I could teach social science in high school, I'll never know. The first time I had to present a lesson, I almost died. The supervisor said he would be gone for an hour and I was to take over until he got back. I literally didn't think I had enough words to keep going for an hour. Looking back, I realize that I never was one to do much talking—even when we had bull sessions in the dorm. I guess I'm what is known as a good conversationalist—I listen and let someone else do the talking. I don't think I've ever talked for more than five minutes at a time, counting my speech classes. It's not that I'm afraid to talk, it's just that I don't want to bore anyone.

Filibuster devices such as "and," "uh," "er," and "um" and others of the same ilk are not unique to stutterers. On the contrary, their very presence in the speech of a youngster who stutters can be accounted for in the same way as in the speech of a normal speaker. Society tolerates a certain number of these stallers in normal speech, but sometimes they exceed even the normal limits for the so-called normal speaker, as is indicated in the following report from a young adult stutterer.

> One of my professors averages twenty "and uh's" and "er um's" per minute for fifty minutes of his boring lectures. I don't think he ever completed a sentence to boot. I don't know how he thinks I can take notes in class if he can't remember how he starts his sentences. Yet, when I've talked to him in the hall after class he doesn't use any of this junk and I'm positive he feels sorry for me because I stutter.

Some Indian tribes not only do not have a word for stuttering, but their speakers do not find it necessary to use filibuster devices when they are talking. Dr. Francis Haines, an authority on Nez Percé Indians, related the following incident to one of the authors. This is part of his account of the conduct of a tribal meeting:

> When the elderly chief paused for several seconds to think of what he was to say next, several people in the audience said "Ah." (Indians don't say "ugh.") Then he continued for several minutes until he paused for an even longer time. No one appeared restless, but again scattered "Ah's" could be heard from the audience. This went on until he sat down to a great chorus of "Ah."

The point illustrated here is that in the Nez Percé culture, the audience signals to the speaker that he still has the floor, instead of as in our culture where the speaker finds he must keep his vocal apparatus signalling—"so," "that is," "er," "and er"—while he tries to think of what he wants to say next. Whereas it might be pleasant to live in an interruption-free culture such as this, we must recognize that it is easier to change the child than the culture in which he lives, especially when the culture is more tolerant of the disrupter than the disrupted.

The child who stutters needs to be tough enough to withstand the disrupting influences and pressures of competitive interrupters, inattentive audiences, or impatient auditors. If he isn't tough enough, his tolerance threshold needs to be raised. He must learn to be able to resist and not break down readily under these pressures. The use of desensitization techniques provides an excellent

means of helping a child raise his tolerance threshold and toughen-
ing him to the rough and tumble of "ordinary" conversations.

### Desensitization Therapy

This approach, credited to Egland and described by Van Riper
(5:371-73), is of value to children in both Phases One and Two.
The child need not know what is going on except that he and
the speech therapist are playing. According to Van Riper, a social
relationship is established with the child. They may be setting up
a toy railroad or some other similar activity. The therapist then
gets the child to talk fluently. This is called the *basal fluency level.*

> This may in rare cases have to begin with grunts or interjections,
> but usually it consists of simple statements of fact, requests, ob-
> servations, etc. The therapist, as he works, thinks aloud in snatches
> of self-talk, commenting on his activity. Soon the child will begin
> to do the same, and by appropriately altering the communicative
> conditions, and his own manner, the therapist gets the child to speak
> with complete fluency (5:372).

Once the child *feels* the basal fluency level, the' therapist then
begins to pressure the child. He may begin to hurry him faster
and faster. But, the important thing, according to Van Riper, is
that when the child's speech begins to break down—he speaks of
impending nonfluency—the therapist should let up on the pressure
and permit the child to return to the basal fluency level. The
signs of impending breakdown can be determined through experience and training but Van Riper points out that just before the
breakdown appears the child's mobility decreases ". . . he freezes,
or his general body movements become jerkier, or the tempo of
his speech changes."

Once the child returns to the basal fluency level, he again is
subjected to pressures until the child *almost* becomes disfluent
again. Van Riper suggests that children do not seem to profit
from more than four of these "pushes" per session. The criterion
for successful accomplishment is that the child remains fluent
throughout the sessions.

The therapist will find that many means are available to permit
a child to talk fluently. This is a partial list of approaches that
help fluency. Others can be added.

The first words of an answer to a question can be provided.

"You say you live at one? Four? . . . Oh yes! 1493 Elmwood Drive. . . . How old are you—six or seven?"

A child often can recite familiar lists such as the names of his brothers and sisters, days of the week, months, numbers. "Tell me the days of the week." (Just as he is about to respond say, "beginning with Sunday.")

A child can rhyme successfully—some can read orally without trouble.

"Tell me what you see in this picture. . . . Yes, that boy is on a boat . . . what's he . . . he's fishing. . . . Has he caught any? . . . How many? One-two-three— You say five. I count only four. Let's try it together."

Sometimes it helps to echo his speech. "You went into the barn, yes and . . . three little pigs and a big fat mother pig."

According to Robinson, parents may be brought into this type of therapy for three reasons: (a) to reveal disruptors which they themselves impose upon the child, (b) to provide a controlled situation for observing clearly the effects of various disruptors upon the child's speech, and (c) to take part in the later stages of therapy, when it becomes important to strengthen gains and adapt the child to disrupting conditions in more customary situations (3:719).

When fluency is firmly established in the therapy session, and when a relationship has been established that permits a child to be confident of the therapist's good intentions, the therapist may act out the role of the oral aggressor. The child may be encouraged, good humoredly, to see if he can resist the therapist's attempts to interrupt or to confuse him. The child and the therapist can read together, one reading one thing, one another. Reading together in a choral setting will not only permit a child to feel his "mouth" working well, but if one of the members drags or speeds up, others in the group can learn to resist this and carry on using their own preconceived appropriate rate.

Several approaches will help a child to spot an inappropriate "uh, uh," or "and," etc., which crop up in his speech. For example, a tape recording can be made of the child relating some interesting experience; while his voice is being recorded, his therapist can add up under separate columns on a sheet of paper the number of "and ah's," "um's," or whatever typical excrescence he uses. When the recording is played back to him, the child makes his own tally, then the two separate findings are compared. This will not only permit him to criticize himself, but it will permit him to take responsibility for his own actions without fear of the penalty which would result if the therapist alone made the judgment. The therapist can make his tally incomplete, so that the balance of criticism will be on the child's side. He can then ask the child to retell the story, trying to keep out a significant number of his stallers. Next, and if he can accept it in a spirit of fun, he can be encouraged to penalize himself by going all the way back to the beginning of his story when he slips up.

> CAUTION: Remember that his history of hesitation may have started because his audience was hypersensitive to his verbal faults. If you suspect that he interprets your efforts as fault-finding, change your tactics. Do something else. However, keep in mind that some of these devices are miniature avoidances, a kind of underbrush that will eventually have to be cleared away if it becomes necessary to work directly on actual moments of stuttering.

### Assuring Successful Opportunities to Talk

The phenomenon of adaptation (the decrease in the average amount of stuttering with successive readings or speaking of the same material) can be used to advantage to modify stuttering. Adaptation points to a significant feature of stuttering—the more the stutterer talks, the less he stutters. The stuttering child should talk as much as possible under as many different conditions as possible.

In the days of the little red schoolhouse, it was not an unusual practice to excuse a stuttering child from recitations. This sometimes happens in today's schools. The teacher gives the excuse that the child is saved from the embarrassment of standing in front of the others to recite. These children may not be embarrassed at all about their stuttering, at least not enough to permit themselves to be treated differently from the other children in their classroom. Many of these children, in fact, learn to be embarrassed through the reactions of their teachers. The embarrassment saved may have been the teacher's.

> One child we knew was prevented from joining choral singing and reading on the grounds that he might stutter. Since the choral activity was compulsory in this school, the child was instructed just to move his lips in time with the others but to utter no sound. It is revealing that when the child was brought to the clinic for

help on his stuttering, his first question was, "Will you please teach me how to sing and read in unison?"

The stuttering child must talk. For the stuttering child silence breeds anxiety. As Sheehan states, "Speaking holds the promise of communication but the threat of stuttering; silence eliminates temporarily the threat involved in speaking, but at a cost of abandonment of communication and consequent frustration. Many stutterers show a *fear of silence* [italics his], and filibuster furiously in their speech to keep any pause from becoming dangerously long. Since most stuttering occurs initially, then silence plus initiation of speech becomes a conditioned cue for the painful experiences of anxiety and stuttering " (4:127).

It is important to know how much a child talks. His reluctance to talk may be a result of his stuttering, but he may also be reluctant because he doesn't have an opportunity to talk, doesn't know what to talk about, or isn't successful in expressing his ideas.

One way to measure a child's concern about the way he talks is to note how much he refrains from talking. A child's shyness can often be offset by providing ample allowance for him to talk about the things he knows well, does well, or even more important, *likes* to talk about. "What should we talk about?" provides a keynote for therapy at this level. This is the kind of encouragement he needs and he should get a lot of it.

This kind of approach sometimes needs to be discussed with the child's parents and teachers because they may be shocked when, in reply to their question, "What do you do when you go out of the room with your speech therapist?" the child blandly replies, "We just talk."

The importance of this approach should be carefully explained to the child's parents and teachers to offset any feelings they may have that this is not a profitable way to spend time out of the classroom. If possible, the parents should be allowed to observe a therapy session in which the therapist uses an approach which he has previously explained to them. Ample allowance for talking during therapy allows the child to speak unhampered by some of the counterpressures to fluency he cannot cope with at home or at school. If the therapist is a permissive listener, the child may finally have a chance to hear himself without the need to be concerned about what he hears. This is a time, too, when he can learn to think on his feet, organize his ideas, and express himself freely. It may be that all he needs is an outlet for his speech. "Just talking," however, can be an opportunity for the therapist to shape quality as well as an opportunity to provide for quantity. The child often construes desensitization therapy as a time when he just talks.*

Actually, no avenue of successful oral performance for the normal speaking child should be closed to the stuttering child. At all stages of stuttering the child needs, and will profit from, the rewarding experience of being exposed to a receptive audience. Classroom projects and activities involving speech are especially good if they permit the expression of newly learned knowledge and provide protection from the onslaughts of interrupters and interruptions.

Since all avenues for successful oral performance should be incorporated into an active therapy program, the stuttering child should be given parts in plays and skits in his classroom, small parts at first, but major parts as he profits from successful participation. One third grader finally blossomed out and became an active participant in all classroom activities because he was cast in the role of a cow in a puppet show about "Jack and The Beanstalk." All he had to say was "moo," but he milked that role for all it was worth.

There is no reason to discourage a child from seeking a leadership role in his class because he stutters. His political desirability may even be enhanced by his limited loquacity. Frequent oral reading sessions (if he can read well) and the recital of poems and stories (if he can do so without having his intelligence impugned or his morale undermined) permit a child to feel a free flow of words without the constraints imposed by trying to grope among many words to express himself.

---

* Some children need special encouragement. Suggestions for encouraging talking can be found in an exemplary book by Charles Van Riper and Katherine G. Butler entitled *Speech in the Elementary Classroom*. Chapter Two of this book deals with improved methods for dealing with sharing time, creative dramatics, group planning and reports, group problem solving, and others. Van Riper and Butler contend that children need more than an *opportunity* to develop speech skills. They need to experiment with actual speech experiences and this excellent little book provides workable measures for successful child-centered experiments in talking.

Charles Van Riper and Katherine G. Butler, *Speech in the Elementary Classroom* (New York: Harper & Row, Publishers, 1955).

*Speech Patterns*

An unconcerned free flow of words is an important aspect of the over-all goal of general speech improvement. Speaking in rhythms, choral speaking, interpretative reading, and any other means of producing free speech flow minimize the chances that awkward silences will become permanent fixtures of a child's speech pattern. The engrams for speech in the brain of a child who stutters are not the engrams of a child whose speech flows gently like sweet Afton. A child with a history of stuttering may, at times, have speech that flows serenely as a meadow stream. But, more often the speech is pent up and pulsing, tumbling as the waters in a twisting, narrow mountain canyon. Sometimes the speech of a child courses rapidly, with the words tumbling over each other; moments later this rapid flow may be dammed up and even stop and start fitfully. As long as the flow is dammed up, the potentially destructive energy continues to build.

The attainment of a free flow of appropriately phrased good speech should be encouraged. A child must learn how to direct his speaking energies into well-worn appropriate channels so as to circumvent the emotional explosions that are bound to occur if his speech is thwarted and cannot move smoothly in its forward course. There are several ways that this can be done.

He should have frequent opportunities to listen to the speech of good speakers. Choral speaking permits him to imitate and echo adequate patterns of well-integrated speaking. If it is inconvenient to have him meet with others for choral speaking purposes, tape recordings of the voices of good speakers can serve as excellent substitutes for live voices. If his speech flows freely without jerks and repetitions on certain days, recordings should be made and saved so that he can echo his own free-flowing speech to refresh his memories of optimal muscle balance and freedom from repetitions, etc. If such recordings are difficult to obtain because his phrasing is chronically awkward, earphones from a public speaking amplifier or desk model hearing aid may be placed on his ears so that he hears only the voice of the therapist as they read the same passage in chorus and record it. If the therapist keeps his voice low enough and stays far enough away as they speak into the microphone, only the child's voice will be recorded. This recording will provide him with examples of adequate speech patterns to echo and imitate.

### Fortifying and Enhancing the Child's Sense of Worth and General Well-Being

How the child feels about himself during therapy and his self-concept afterward are major considerations in any plan of therapy. A stutterer whose mediocre skills and talents are relatively unrewarded stands much less chance of improving than the stutterer who has compensating talents and receives rewards of achievement, acknowledgment, and praise. The speech therapist must be careful not to place all the focus on the way the child talks. A well-balanced program will allow time for finding and nourishing those things that a child can do well whether it be reading, singing, climbing a tree, or spinning a yo-yo "around the world." Therapy for a child in any stage of stuttering should provide for a careful inventory of his assets and liabilities so that the therapist can bring the child to a self-concept of strong pride in his own worth.

Insecurity may stem from sources less obvious than stuttered speech. Questioning the child's parents and teachers should give clues to unusual fears or anxieties. Special tests measure his sight, hearing, and academic achievement. His oral reading may be poor because his silent reading skills are poor, or because he cannot see or hear well. His health, his intelligence, his performance in arithmetic and spelling may all affect his feelings of security. When correctable deficiencies are uncovered remedial programs other than speech are indicated and may even supersede speech therapy aimed at improved intelligibility and corrected misarticulations.

### Honesty Is the Best Policy

To ignore the fact that a child is having difficulty in talking is helpful when the child is unaware that his way of talking is different from others. But, as stated earlier, children at the Phase Two level are aware of their stuttering and often call it "stuttering." In the section of this chapter concerned with counseling parents, the point was made that ignoring stuttering at this stage may increase rather than decrease the child's problem. The same point applies to the therapist. Children at this level of stuttering may need a more directive approach. Some of them, in fact, will probably appreciate the opportunity to talk about their problem. It is well to remember that the amount of stuttering a child displays may not correlate with his feelings about it. A child may show only little stuttering and be deeply concerned, or he may have speech that is marked by frequent moments of stuttering and only be intrigued—not disturbed—by the way he sounds.

In those cases where the child shows awareness of his problem and where the therapist senses a desire on the part of the child to bring the problem up for discussion, the therapist need not be afraid to talk directly with him about the difficulty he is having. These discussions need not, and probably should not, be as directive as those with a Phase Three or Phase Four stutterer, but they still can deal directly with the child's stuttering and his feelings about speaking. The basic attitude the therapist should demonstrate during these discussions is that *he* is not deeply concerned about the way the child talks, but he is concerned about the way the child *feels* about the way he talks. The therapist shows that he is willing to listen and to help.

If the child complains that his speech is different, the therapist will probably accomplish little by protesting immediately that it isn't. Too much protestation on the therapist's part may force the child into unnecessary, complicated justifications of his feelings. There will be time later to rebuild his confidence in his speaking ability. At this moment the therapist needs to listen and accept the child's problem—to avoid contradicting his judgment. Such a child as we now have in mind probably knows that something unusual is going on in his speech. To help him maintain his self-respect, it may be best to let him struggle with his own courage and respect his right to test his own anxiety. He may wonder what these repetitions and bobbles are leading to. He may be afraid that he will lose completely his ability to talk. The therapist can provide reassurance, but this is most effective after the child decides that the therapist understands him and his problem.

Since most stutterers at this level show little concern over their stuttering, the therapist will want to avoid the type of reassuring remark that suggests deeper feelings than exist, such as, "I understand what you must be going through," said in a pitying manner. There are times, though, when these children do feel sensitive about their perceived inability to "speak right." If the occasion arises, the therapist may point out that many children feel pretty low and discouraged when they think their speech is unacceptable. At times, they may even feel like crying. If the child indicates that he does not want to talk at all in some circumstances, the therapist can accept this feeling and even point out that it is not unreasonable to feel this way when the going gets rough. When the therapist feels that most of the child's problem is talked out, it is legitimate and even vitally important to suggest that things will turn out well. One reason a child sometimes brings up such problems is to hear from the lips of someone he respects that he will improve. Reassurances to this effect need not be exaggerated, but he may be shown that his speech musculature is capable of producing fluent speech, that he does speak fluently more often than not, and that in the therapist he has someone who is willing to continue talking with him until he feels better about the problem.

With some Phase Two stutterers, methods for modifying their typical attempts to say difficult words can be taught. Techniques for decreasing tension in the articulators (essentially the same as the loose contacts suggested for more advanced stutterers) can be taught but in a very indirect manner. The therapist may show the child how he can say difficult words by consciously loosening up the tension on his lips or tongue. He can be shown how the muscles around the lips operate like the drawstring on mother's purse or the top of his pajamas—the tighter he pulls the string, the smaller the opening. He can learn to feel the difference in his lips when pushing hard on words like "papa" or "baby" and when puffing these same beginning sounds lightly through his lips. The same principles can be applied to words where the tongue or vocal folds are involved. He may learn that his tendency to "get stuck" is more likely to happen when he is upset, excited, or anxious, and he may even learn to recognize and guard against those conditions which increase his tension.

Even though relatively direct measures are employed at times, with the Phase Two stutterer it is important to remember that the child's concept of being different is not strongly fixed and that the stuttering has a good chance of disappearing under proper management. Discussions about feelings and suggestions for modifying speech should not be made in such a way as to imply that the problem is permanent.

### The Story of Mike—a Phase Two Stutterer

This history of one child's stuttering is described through his mother's letters to the speech therapist. This is not presented as an example of an ideal therapy situation—for it was not—nor even of ideal therapeutic management, but it illustrates well life's ups and downs and their effect upon stuttering. The reader is urged to notice the many different environmental factors that were related to the fluctuations in stuttering.

Attention should be directed also to the difficulties in classifying stuttering as to level of development. In many respects, Mike's stuttering might better be classified as Phase Three or, at times, as Phase Four. The struggle behavior noted in the mother's call on February 29, the use of postponements mentioned in the May 27 letter, and the avoidance behavior in the filmed interview of January 12 all suggest a more advanced classification of stuttering. On the other hand, Mike's willingness to continue talking, his frequent periods of little or no stuttering, and his general tendency to display relatively easy repetitions and prolongations without apparent avoidance and emotional reaction lead to a classification of Phase Two stuttering.

Because of space, notes concerning what took place during his clinic visits are not included except where it helps to maintain the continuity of the letters. Several letters and visits to the clinic have not been included.


February 5    Clinic Files

Both mother and father visited the speech and hearing center with Mike during the first visit. Both parents are from Oklahoma —father is a slow deliberate talker—mother claims to be and is a fast talker. Parents intelligent and alert. Father supervisor at metal plant. Mother works as private secretary. Mike has one older brother. Mike not always able to compete with him successfully. Mike has an uncle in Oklahoma who stutters. There was one time when three families lived in the same house—Mike's Aunt's family, the maternal grandparents, and Mike's family. Little niece teased Mike unmercifully. At present time Mike's brother and neighbor child tease Mike about his stuttering and call him baby.

Mike, a first grader, repeats words and prolongs the initial sounds of some words. He refers to his way of talking as stuttering.

Early talker. Enough disfluency to be concerned about. Sharp youngster. Talks considerably. In fact parents report that he talks all the time. They live too far away for regular visits to the center. . . .

Suggestions made to parents concerning ways to handle stuttering at home. Explanation of nature of stuttering given. Discussed problem of teasing. Temporary therapy plan to center around helping parents know how to handle problem. Mother was requested to write once a month about the status of his speech. Made appointment for March 9.

February 29    Clinic Files

Mother called on the 29th of February and said that she hadn't written but had become concerned because the boy had begun to toss his head, etc., while stuttering. An appointment was made for the next day instead of waiting until March 9.

March 1    Clinic Files

Father is now working graveyard shift and is sleeping during the day. The trouble began about last week on Monday or Tuesday, and Saturday and Sunday this past week have been especially rough on the boy because he had trouble being quiet while father was sleeping. Mother took both boys away from home on Sunday so that father could sleep. Father, according to Mother, has been bending over backwards to avoid being cranky with the children. Things have been complicated because the sister's daughter, the niece who teases Mike, showed up Tuesday or Wednesday. Although she was only there about 45 minutes, mother thinks this may have had some effect on Mike's speech. Also he had one tooth filled and one pulled and is having some trouble wearing the spacer in his lower jaw.

Took Mike to the group room and talked with him about his stuttering. Mike didn't seem to be too disturbed about it. Showed him how to let up on the forcing when it occurred and explained how struggling makes it harder to say words. Showed him how he could stutter on purpose but without struggling. Reinforced the idea that it was important to keep on talking. Checked to find out who some of the boys were who teased him at school. Talked about how he felt about this and what he could do to handle it.

Mother is to write every week now until the stuttering seems to abate. Mike doesn't seem to be too disturbed about the stuttering. Emphasized to mother that she should not attempt to repress the stuttering, talk about it to him, etc. . . .

March 7

DEAR SIR:

Since we were up there last Tuesday Mike hasn't improved too much. He tried to show me how to stutter. He had me count from one to ten just like you did with him and he kept asking me which stutter was real and which was pretend. We got along pretty good.

I called his teacher when we got home Tuesday, and she had had a conference cancellation so I went on over to the school and we had his conference. The mothers of the children Mike named as the ones who teased him hadn't been in for their conference yet so she said she would talk to them about it. Also it was decided that maybe she should change their seats around since those three little boys had Mike surrounded in the seating arrangement. She was very glad to get the little book and immediately noticed the section on "Crutches" so I went ahead and explained to her why it was better not to encourage that sort of thing.

His teacher suggested that to stop the teasing at school maybe Mike could just tell the class all about it and about you, but I told her that I didn't think we should until we had talked it over with you. What is your opinion on this?

Mike has been sleeping well and eating like a pig. He did have some trouble last week. He developed a boil or something similar to one on his arm. We've whipped that now so it isn't bothering him any more. Friday he got hit in the head with a fire extinguisher at school and came home with a big lump on his forehead.

I'll keep an eye on Mike this week and will call you later in the week if he doesn't improve.

March 8

DEAR MRS.———:

Why couldn't his teacher talk to the entire class while Mike is out of the room on some pretext. This might help considerably, especially if she pointed out that she did not want to hear of any more reference to the way he talked. Ask her to stress that it is more important to listen to *what* he says rather than to *how* he says it. I don't think that Mike is sophisticated enough or objective enough at this time to talk to the entire group about his stuttering. The solution concerning the seating arrangement is a good one. . . .

March 17

DEAR SIR:

There's not much to report this time. Mike seems to have improved a little bit. Spring vacation from school has helped a little. Last week he protested against having to eat a hot lunch at school. Also he refused to ride the school bus home in the afternoon. Instead he walked the eleven blocks regardless of weather. There must be something going on in the lunch room and on the bus but that's something we can't do too much about. I let him take a sack lunch every day, so we eliminated the cafeteria problem for last week, anyway.

Mike and his dad are old buddy-buddies this week and so Dad has become a very important character. They are redoing Mike's bicycle—new paint, new seat, etc. But we have this graveyard shift facing us the end of next week. So we'll see what happens to Mike's speech then.

He hasn't been having any severe blocks the last few days but last week when he would have a block and I would mention it to him he would take several deep breaths and then be able to talk OK. I didn't know whether this was a suggestion from you* or something he had worked out for himself.

If he refuses to eat at the cafeteria next week and walks home from school, I don't know what we'll do. I'll write you again as soon as we see how Mike reacts to graveyard shift next week.

March 30

DEAR SIR:

We'll have to call this a "progress report" this time. Mike has improved quite a bit these last ten days. Graveyard shift hasn't bothered him too much. He had a busy weekend so wasn't home too much of the time. There was a birthday party Saturday after-

---

* It wasn't.

noon and Sunday School Sunday morning so that time away from home relieved the strain.

I don't know what happened at school Monday but he was sort of flustered when he got home, and had difficulty all evening but seems to have straightened out some.

But now we are faced with a new situation. Big brother all but broke his foot at school yesterday. Has no broken bones but lots of torn and bruised ligaments in the top of his foot. Can't go to school for a week and then will be in a cast and on crutches for three weeks. All this has taken the limelight away from Mike. He seems to resent most of all that Bobby gets to stay home from school while he has to go. He raised quite a fuss this morning. We'll just have to wait a while and see how he adjusts to all this before I take any drastic measures.

I haven't seen his teacher in quite a while but if Mike was having any trouble at school I think she would have called me.

That's about all there is to report this time. I will write again if anything happens.


April 18

DEAR SIR:

I wrote you one letter last week but didn't get it mailed. I was real worried about Mike. He got up on Sunday morning and was getting ready for Sunday School and could scarcely get a word out. He was still stuttering badly when he got back home, so I wrote you but before I could get it mailed he had straightened up and could talk again without any hesitation. Now he seems to have reached a plateau and leveled off and there hasn't been any radical change. He isn't as bad as he was when we were at your office the last time but there is still room for improvement. He has rare moments when he has trouble but they are getting farther apart.

I talked to his teacher and she says that he has improved at school, too. Now when he tells things he doesn't get as tangled up as he used to. And the kids all sit patiently waiting for him to finish. She says that he still tells long involved stories but they don't seem so long to the kids because he doesn't stutter like he did. I think his trouble that Sunday morning was that it was the first time he had gone to Sunday School by himself. Big brother couldn't go because of his foot. He went this Sunday again alone and it didn't upset him at all. Apparently he has his confidence back now.

My job opens up the end of next month and I'll be going back to work. I worked last fall from the time Mike started to school until the end of November. Then again in January for three weeks. I don't know what effect this had on Mike, but we'll soon see if it had anything to do with his trouble becoming worse. I don't think it has anything to do with it. He became very self-sufficient during that time and seemed to enjoy being on his own. I'll keep you posted on how he reacts this time.


May 27

DEAR SIR:

I guess it is about time that I wrote you again. And I have a bad report to make this time. Mike has started to stutter again. There for quite a while things seemed to maintain a status quo but for the last couple of weeks his stuttering has become progressively worse. No doubt, he has something bothering him, but I don't know what it is. There are a few things that he could be worried about.

Big brother's foot is back to normal and he doesn't seem to be giving Mike a hard time. I have been watchful about this and can discern no noticeable change in their relationship. He may have become upset over something at school. He had a nosebleed at school the other day and he wasn't hit, so he must have gotten excited about something. He wouldn't talk about it when he got home except to explain about the blood on his shirt and assure me that no one hit him. I have been working three or four days a week and Mike has been baby-sitting himself for an hour a day after school but I don't think that has upset him. He loves the added independence that this affords him. If there is something he wants to do that he thinks I may not approve of he always calls me at work so I can tell him "no." He is a very independent little boy anyway and loves to be more or less his own boss for that hour between the time he gets home and the time that big brother arrives.

Also, he is forming the habit of using "uh" an awful lot. Almost every other word is "uh." He hesitates over his words and the "uh" just naturally comes out while he is apparently trying to think of the next one. There are so many things that could be bothering him that I have no way of ever discovering. So we will just have to consider what we do know. . . .

May 31    Clinic Files

Talked to mother on the phone concerning her letter of May 27. Father was on graveyard shift when Mike's symptoms worsened, but now he is on the day shift again. The grunting continues. Asked her whether the termination of school has some bearing and she feels this might be a possibility. Also, a relative's child from Idaho arrived last night. He is seven or eight months older than Mike and apparently they quarreled all evening. They are working out some adjustment for this. Mother will be in with Mike on June 7 at 11:00.

June 7    Clinic Files

Visit to center. Very little hesitation. Some "uh" between words as reported by mother. Mike talks readily about his stuttering.

July 13

DEAR SIR:

I have finally found a few minutes in which to write you, and I have good news this time. Mike has almost entirely quit stuttering. There has been a remarkable improvement in his speech since school let out. He has finally oriented himself to all of his free time and doesn't try to crowd all of his playing into one day. So, consequently he doesn't get as tired as he was for a while. The only time he has trouble talking is when he has done something he shouldn't and is having to explain his actions in such a way as to prove himself in the right. His stuttering then comes from not being able to think fast enough. The last talk I had with his teacher she said she thought Mike should read some this summer if he wanted to but that text books weren't permitted to leave the school so I would have to get Mike a library card and use their books. But I've been working five and one-half days a week and haven't had time to obtain one for him. I noticed him last week, though, reading an old reader that I had when I was in the first grade. So he hasn't lost his interest in reading.

Dad is getting ready to start graveyard shift again and that may affect Mike but there is a promise of a camping trip on the 21st so that may sustain Mike through graveyard shift and the trial of having Dad sleeping in the daytime. If there is any new development I'll let you know immediately.

August 10
DEAR SIR:

I decided I had better write again. Mike is off and running. He has started to stutter again quite badly. And, boy, does he ever have reason to this time.

He has poison oak till it has about driven him crazy. For a week he had had it all over his penis and surrounding area. He didn't sleep at night and neither did I. The doctor had him on cortisone pills, ACTH shots, wetpacks, sedatives, and anti-itch pills of some sort. And there was cortisone ointment to rub on. He was a nervous wreck when it finally began to clear up. He now has an infected finger and has a doctor's appointment for today. Looks like it will have to be lanced. He's real worried about his finger of course; it is painful. Yesterday a little neighbor boy hit him right in the middle of the forehead and now he is sporting a big knot and bruise. The weapon the kid used was a lead pipe. Mike sure has had a rough summer!

I've been working but he hasn't had to stay with a baby sitter. His grandpa has been coming over every day and either they stay home with him or he takes them somewhere.

Mike's nerves are shot from just having one thing after the other. He is getting so irritable we can hardly live with him. Whines quite a bit and talks baby talk a lot. He had a birthday August 1 and was disappointed to not have a party this year. We had a big one last year. But we had a fancy cake from the bakery.

No one has been riding Mike about his stuttering this time. Everyone knows of his circumstances and we have all been very patient with him. But I don't quite know how to handle this baby talk thing. Maybe it will just go away. I surely hope so. If you have suggestions on how to handle this situation I would appreciate hearing them. Maybe if we could get all his ailments cured at one time and his nerves could settle down then the stuttering will take care of itself. . . .

September 15
DEAR SIR:

I guess it is about time to report in again. Mike's finger cleared up as did his poison oak. And school has started. He is still stuttering but not as badly as he was when he had his poison oak and infected finger at the same time.

Starting back to school didn't upset him at all that I could tell. He has the same teacher that he had last year so we won't have to go through breaking in a new teacher to all of Mike's little peculiarities. I guess that is something to be thankful for.

I haven't talked to his teacher yet as to how Mike is doing in school. It is a little too soon to tell yet about his school work but she should be able to tell me if he stutters at school. Of course, the only time that I see him is in the evening when he is tired and I know that he usually stutters then. He doesn't do too much in the morning before school. I guess the best thing to do would be to let it rock along until I can see his teacher and find out what he does at school.

Right now Mike doesn't have anything physically wrong with him and as soon as he gets used to the routine of school again he will settle down, we hope. So I will write you again in a couple of weeks and in the meantime I will make a point of seeing his teacher. . . .


Appointment was made to see Mike in the Speech and Hearing Center:


September 28    Clinic Files

Talked with Mike for a short time today. His speech apparently does fluctuate considerably. Difficult to make an adequate judgment from the small sample heard. Did hear occasional short repetitions of syllables. Mother claims he was entirely fluent all the way over in the car and that he talked a "blue streak" without any stuttering. . . .


October 19
DEAR SIR:

It's about time that I report on Mike again. He seems to be about status quo. He seems to be some better than he was when I brought him up to see you. He and his father and brother went on a three-day hunting trip this past weekend. It was a tiring trip for the little fellow. They drove over a thousand miles. Went way over in Eastern Oregon on the Snake River. Mainly it was a scouting trip for big elk hunt later this month but the boys thought it was a deer hunting trip for them.

His Dad was telling me about a bad experience that Mike had in a cafe that they stopped in. Said that it embarrassed Mike and him and the waitress. Whenever we take the kids to a cafe they always do their own ordering and this time when it came Mike's turn he had one of those blocks that we have discussed. He had been chattering right along up 'till the time that it came his turn to order and I guess the fact that he was in the spotlight gave him stage fright and he had this block and couldn't tell the waitress what he wanted. His father said that he started over and over again and would get to one certain point and couldn't go any farther. He finally started to cry and so his father told the waitress to just go ahead with what he and brother had ordered and when Mike made up his mind he would tell her. After she was gone Mike settled down and told his Dad all he wanted was a tuna fish sandwich. I don't know whether it was the waitress that upset him or maybe it was the fact that ordinarily he hates tuna fish sandwiches and wouldn't touch one of them at home. Usually all that Mike will order in a cafe is a dish of ice cream. Maybe a major change over from ice cream to tuna fish was too difficult a decision for him to make.

Anyway, it is over and past and Mike didn't even mention it to me. But it was a block. He was forcing too much and his tongue was locked in the roof of his mouth and he just couldn't say what he had in mind.

Outside of this one incident, Mike has been doing fine. He has had his one cold of the season and doesn't seem to be stuttering any worse than he was when you talked to him. I'll be reporting in again in a few weeks or sooner if anything comes up. . . .


December 29
DEAR SIR:

It has been a long time, hasn't it? And it must be time for another progress report. Sorry I can't call this one a "progress report." But Mike has leveled off on this one plane and doesn't get any better.

Since the last time I wrote you—I believe I have written you since he started on this last binge—he reached his low level and stuttered real badly and we have been waiting and waiting for him to pull out of it and make some progress but he just doesn't make enough so that I can feel that he is reaching that high level like he used to.

The excitement of Christmas and the prospect of getting a new bicycle could have been a contributing factor to holding him down. He got the bicycle Christmas morning and was real thrilled over it. But you remember how it rained. It was two days before he could take it out. He jumped on, rolled down the drive, fell off and put his feet through the spokes. The bike is still rideable but he was one disappointed boy. He hasn't gotten as much rest as he should during this vacation from school and that could have a lot to do with it also. I'm pretty sure he hasn't had trouble at school or his teacher would have called me.

So, it is anybody's guess as to what is holding him down. But he hasn't pulled out of this low level like he should have to conform to this pattern he has set for himself.


January 5    Clinic Files

An appointment was made to see Mike's mother in the center and to discuss these problems and at the same time to make some more motion pictures of Mike. These pictures were being taken from time to time as a record of his speech.


January 12    Clinic Files

Came in to make the motion picture. According to mother he has become a "stinker"—gripes at mother—says, "goodbye mean mama." Cries easily at school—he doesn't get hurt physically—not enough to cry, but he cries. Is in bed at 8:30 doesn't get to sleep until 9:30. Was flicking his hand and jerking his head as release, but stopped when mother said "did you hurt your hand? Are you drying your finger nails?" Mike gets better every time mother tells him he is coming to the clinic. He quit stuttering when she got the letter with the appointment on the 7th.

The following is excerpted from the movie sound track taken that day. The conversation is similar in content to sessions during his infrequent visits to the speech clinic.

Interviewer: Mike you say you've been having trouble with your speech?

Mike: Well, wh-when I'm talking—sometimes I get, uh, sometimes I get stuck on a word and say it over and over again.

Int.: You keep saying it over and over? Do you ever get to the point where you can't say it at all?

Mike: Uh, uh no!

Int.: You can usually say it, huh? How does it sound when you say it over and over again?

Mike: Well, uh, it, uh, sounds something like this. Wh-wh-wh-when I, I say something, well, it sounds something like this kind of stuff.

Int.: Uh huh, you can do this "stuff" on purpose. What do you call this "stuff"?

Mike: Stuttering.

Int.: You call this stuttering then.

Mike: Yes.

Int.: And you can do it on purpose can you?

Mike: Yes.

Int.: Let me hear some of it. What did you get for Christmas? See if you can do some of that on purpose as you tell me.

Mike: Well, I, I, I got a guhgun and I got a buhbuhbike.

Int.: Was that real?

Mike: No.

Int.: You made believe there? Huh?

Mike: Yes.

Int.: But you said that you never get stuck and hung up so bad you can't say it at all? Do you ever have words that almost get stuck?

Mike: Uh huh!

Int.: What do you do then?

Mike: Well, I stop a minute and then, uh, I start over and then I can talk through sometimes.

Int.: Do you sometimes try to find another word?

Mike: Yeah, if there is one word I get stuck on. Well, I, I pick another word that means the same thing.

Int.: Do you do that a lot?

Mike: Some—yeah!

Int.: What usually happens? Do you have to find another word or do you stop and wait 'till you're over it or do you juhjuhjust keep on repeating the word?

Mike: Sometimes I juhjuhjust keep on repeating the word.

Int.: Well, when you said juhjust, was that one of those times?

Mike: Yeah.

Int.: And you say most of the times you just keep on repeating.

Mike: I, I get stuck, stuck, on, on, uh, uh, w-word when, only when I t-talk f-fast.

Int.: You get stuck when you're talking fast?

Mike: Yes—when I'm excited and when I'm talking fast.

Int.: Now at school do you still have that show and tell time?

Mike: Uh huh.

Int.: What do you do in that?

Mike: Wwwe tell the class about our trip and where we, we've b-been on school days and the days we, we're home and the things we get.

Int.: Oh, do you do that? Do you get up and tell them?

Mike: Yup!

Int.: How often?

Mike: Mmm.

Int.: Every day?

Mike: Not every day, uh, uh, a few days we do that.

Int.: Do you like to share and tell?

Mike: Show and tell!

Int.: Show and tell. Do you like to do that?

Mike: Well, a few times I, I get, I, uh, have trouble. Bu-but most of the time I like to.

Int.: What kind of trouble do you have?

Mike: Stuttering.

Int.: You stutter at those times? Do the other kids notice it?

Mike: Th-they, I, I don't think they even know about it.

Int.: They never mock you or tease you or anything like that?

Mike: Nnno, bu-but in the first grade they knew about it and teased me.

Int.: Can you tell about it?

Mike: We-well they ke-kept ta-taking my ha-hat and sta-started chasing me. Th-they started chasing me around the school grounds.

Int.: Did they say anything to you?

Mike: I, I, I forgot, forgot what they said now but—

Int.: What do you remember?

Mike: Every time they chased me I told the teacher what they were doing and uh, and uh, every time they saw me walking toward, toward the teacher they rrran off so the teacher couldn't tell who they were.

Int.: They ran off but they didn't call you names?

Mike: No!


January 31

DEAR SIR:

Another report on the life and times of Mike. He has been up to his old tricks again. He has had poison oak again. And all over his body. I wish he could just have it on his arm like most other people, but he goes all out. He is just about over it and is back in school. He missed three days last week. He has been on cortisone and tranquilizers. Of course, his stuttering got worse while he was so itchy but I talked to his teacher this morning and he has been doing real well at school. He even gave a talk yesterday to the class about the museum he visited. His Dad took him and brother over there Saturday and then Mike told his class yesterday about all the things he saw. His teacher said that the only time he stuttered was at the beginning of the sentence and then he would just go right on. She listened more to his stuttering than to his story.

The kids in his room had a reading test last Thursday and his teacher was afraid to let Mike take the test his first day back at school and as uncomfortable as he was but he insisted so she let him take it along with the rest of the class. He came out with a raw score of 30 which looked pretty good to me in comparison with some of the others. So he must have felt better than he looked.

Mike really acted like a big wheel when I took him back to school. The kids all ganged around him and were exclaiming over the fact that Mike was back in school. They all wanted to know why he had been absent and instead of just telling them he had poison oak he sat there with his hand on his forehead and looked pathetic and said, "Oh, I've been sick." Then they all felt sorry for him and he was pleased with all the attention he was getting. A real big ham. . . .

He is still stuttering at home but doesn't seem to at school so much. As soon as the aftereffects of this poison oak medicine wears off, then we can tell more about it. Right now he is off the cortisone pills and shots but there is sure to be some still in his bloodstream and he is still jittery. If the cortisone is a cure for arthritis, then Mike will never have it. . . .


March 13

DEAR SIR:

I don't know what to report about Mike. He fluctuates so much from day to day that it is hard to tell just what he is doing. Right now he has an exhibit ready for the science fair. He has made a pulley to enter in the primary division.

Some days he stutters so badly that we can hardly understand him and others he talks just fine. His teacher is still watching him pretty close and lets me know if anything happens at school. Right now he seems to be marking time and not getting anywhere.

But I guess that is to be expected from time to time. We can't expect constant progress.

Say, how would you like to meet Mike's big brother who bugs him so? If I came up Friday I could bring him also. The kids are out of school for spring vacation. If you met this guy maybe then you would know why he bugs Mike.

Anyway, I will call you Thursday and let you know. . . . [And they came in and we met his brother, and he turned out to be like most brothers.]

### April 7   Clinic Files

Mother called because Mike and neighbor boy had washed a neighbor lady's puppy in her automatic washer—the puppy was drowned in the process. Started to stutter severely.

### April 17
Dear Sir:

I don't know exactly how to start this and I would like to see your face while you read it. I guess we can call this another chapter in the "Life of Mike."

The incident of the puppy is forgotten or so it seems. I called Mrs.——— and talked to her about how he acted at school that Friday after it happened. She said he was a little quieter than usual and she didn't have to call him down as often but he and G———, the other boy involved—marched right into school that morning and told her all about it. G——— was more upset over it than Mike and so Mike told the story. But she said it was a very well prepared little story—well thought out ahead of time. Mike scarcely stuttered at all while telling it but he would say a sentence and then stop and swallow and then say another sentence. G——— stuttered so badly she couldn't understand a word he said all day. But, anyway, that was when she got her licks in about how to take care of baby animals. So she had already been through that bit before I could stop her. They haven't mentioned the puppy so apparently it has been pushed into the background now. One thing that came out in their story to her that we hadn't heard before was—the day before they drowned the poor little thing they had put him in my dryer and given him a few fast turns in it, so I'm glad that I spanked him.

There have been new developments since then. Seems like everything happens on Friday. Last Friday, when I got home from work Mike wasn't there. I sent Bobby to find him and he said he was playing in a field a few blocks from the house. The kids have built a back-stop out of some old boards and they play ball down there sometimes. About 5:30 a strange car drove up out in front of the house. There was a man and a little boy in it. Since I didn't recognize the car I didn't look too closely at who was in it. It was parked there for a few minutes and then MIKE jumped out and ran to the house and the man drove off. When Mike came in I began to question him. "Who was the man?" He didn't know. "Why did he bring you home?" He didn't know. "Why did you get into the car with him?" He was walking by the car and the man opened the door and said, "Get in. I'll take you home." So Mike got in. "Did he say anything else to you?" "No. Just that if I ever go down there to play again he'll give me a ride home." "Was he somebody's father?" (Meaning one of his little friends.) Mike said, "Well no, but he was old enough to be a father."

What made it all so fishy was that Mike had ridden his bicycle down there and left it. So I took him down to get his bike and the fellow had gone back there and parked again. There were quite a few little kids playing around there.

So when Dad got up about 6:30 (he is sleeping days now) we talked it over and decided maybe we should call the police. Our town has more than its share of child molesters. So we did— and here came two big burly policemen out to the house. I told them what happened. Can't you just hear in your mind the theme song of "Dragnet"? They talked to Mike and asked questions—lots of questions and hedged all around the one thing they were trying to find out—and Mike stuttered in his most grand and glorious manner. Really much worse than when he drowned the puppy. He was very nervous and on the spot. He had his shirt off and he rolled the front of his undershirt up and down about 50 times. They finally left, telling me that if I ever saw the car again to call them immediately and all sorts of things like that.

They went over and questioned the people who live across the street from this field and they knew who the fellow was, so the police went to see him and that's when the whole story came out. The fellow is a contractor who bought 150 lots including this field and he is going to build houses. He had the foundation in for one and had poured fresh cement that day and Mike had been (so the fellow says) pulling the bolts out of the forms. Mike says he was only hitting the boards with a stick. Well, when they build the house and the foundations give way we'll know why. The police came back and told us what they had found out. So nothing drastically wrong except that Mama and Daddy got excited. I guess the police chewed the man out and told him to not give any more rides to small boys and they told Mike not to get into cars with strange men. He's been told this before but it didn't get through to him. I think probably now he gets the message.

He seems to be bouncing back pretty fast after all of these things. He is pretty well straightened out today but who knows what tomorrow will bring. If this is any indication of what the summer will be like I'm tempted to lock him in his room. I think he was just a little bit pleased at having two big policemen right in our front room but when he heard what they had found out he wasn't too happy then.

I saw an article in the Journal about the stuttering clinic this summer. What Mike needs is a clinic in how to stay out of trouble.

While Mike was dressing this morning he asked me if I would write to you for him and ask if he could come up to see you again. He said he thinks he ought to talk to you again before school is out. What he wants to talk about, I don't know. . . .


June 14
DEAR SIR:

How goes it with you? Everything is pretty quiet at our house. Bobby is going to summer school for advanced kids here in our town and Mike is on his own. Dad has been working graveyard for the last week and sleeping in the daytime. That, at its best, always presents a problem. But Mike has been doing real well. In fact, I think he is surprising himself. Several times in the past two weeks he has said something about how he isn't stuttering much lately.

Did you see the re-run of the Henessey show on television about the boy who stuttered? Mike did. It was his bedtime but I let him stay up and I watched his reaction to the whole thing. He was very much interested and his first reaction was, "Oh that poor sailor stutters." But he sat there and nodded his head to all of the advice that was given this boy. When it was over he said he was sure that the boy could be helped if he would only go to the Clinic because look what it has done for me. So evidently Mike feels that he has made some progress.

We'll soon see what effect having Mother home all of the time will have on him. Tomorrow is my last day of work for a while. Instead of quitting I am taking a leave of absence, for the whole summer, I hope. The boss didn't want me to quit altogether so we are closing the office except for two days a week and the girl from the other office will come over for those days. I'll probably come back to work after school starts again. But in the meantime I can stay home and find out what my kids do when I'm gone.

Mike has had a relatively quiet time accident-wise, too. He has a few minor spots of poison oak on him now but it doesn't bother him very much. Sunday he was jumping up and down in the kitchen and hooked his chin over the edge of the cabinets and almost bit his tongue off. It really did bleed. Other than that he's had a real easy time since school was out.

Of course, he passed the second grade with flying colors. His teacher wrote on his report card that he was very well adjusted in spite of the stuttering. I guess that's good.

I'll let you know if he gets any worse, but right now he is doing as well as can be expected. He does have his moments but for the most part he doesn't stutter at all. He is playing too hard and getting too tired so it may crop out again. I'll let you know because sometimes (and usually) that perks him up and he gets better.


Mike didn't return to the center again. More than a year and one half elapsed before we wrote Mike's mother for her permission to reprint excerpts from some of her letters. Here are some of her comments: Jan 11 ". . . Some of the things I had written about had been forgotten by all of us. . . . Now, it all sounds like a great set-up for a situation comedy series for television. At the time all of that was happening it didn't sound so funny. Thank heavens, he isn't leading that wild kind of life now.

"He had so many things happen to him and he got into so much trouble during that little more than a year that it's no wonder he stuttered. I'm surprised now that he even survived it with all of his senses still at his command. . . . We hope that forever more we can refer to this as Mike's 'toughest year.' I hope he never has to go through that much again, at least in that short space of time."

Signed (Mike's Mother)

*References*

1. BLOODSTEIN, O. "The Development of Stuttering: III—Theoretical and Clinical Implications," *Journal of Speech and Hearing Disorders,* XXVI (1961), 67-82.
2. HULL, C. L. *A Behavior System: An Introduction to Behavior Theory Concerning the Individual Organism* (New Haven: Yale University Press, 1952).
3. ROBINSON, F. "Nature and Treatment of Stuttering in Children," in *Voice and Speech Disorders: Medical Aspects.* N. A. Levin (ed.) (Springfield, Ill.: Charles C. Thomas, 1962).
4. SHEEHAN, J. "Conflict Theory of Stuttering," in *Stuttering: A Symposium,* J. Eisenson (ed.) (New York: Harper & Row, Publishers, 1958).
5. VAN RIPER, C. *Speech Correction: Principles and Methods,* Fourth Ed. (Englewood Cliffs, N.J.: Prentice-Hall, Inc., 1963).
6. WILLIAMS, D. E. "A Point of View about Stuttering," *Journal of Speech and Hearing Disorders,* XXII (1957), 390-97.

*Chapter Five*

## Direct Therapy with Confirmed
## Stutterers (Phase Three)

*At this stage of development symptoms of stuttering are full-fledged except that consistent avoidance of words and situations has not become a habitual reaction to speech. The possessor now is confirmed in his views that his way of talking is a problem and in most cases associated symptoms such as word substitutions, word and sound difficulties, and to a lesser degree conscious anticipations of trouble are present in his speech. Postponement, release, and starting devices are actively employed although they are not firmly established. Outward signs of deep fear or embarrassment are lacking, but the child is deeply aware of his stuttering and direct therapy aimed at associated symptoms and providing an adequate way of attacking difficult words is imperative.*

This chapter discusses the management of stuttering which has progressed to the point where, as far as diagnosis is concerned, the child is obviously in need of speech help. At this stage of development, the stuttering child feels that speaking, for him, is a truly difficult task. Indirection, insofar as reference to the way he talks, is no longer necessary since he views what he does as a personal shortcoming. He is acutely aware that his way of talking is different from that of others and he has had ample confirmation for his convictions through accumulated evidence of difficulty with certain sounds and words or embarrassment while talking.

*Secondary stuttering* is a term commonly used to describe the characteristic symptomatology found in advanced, complex forms of the disorder. Bloodstein describes this developmental stage as Phase Three and differentiates this phase of stuttering from the most advanced form wherein the symptoms of stuttering appear fully developed. The age range of Phase Three stutterers is very wide. Such stutterers may be identified as early as eight years. At the other extreme, they may be found frequently in adulthood, especially milder cases (3).

At this level of stuttering, therapy is direct: the child is involved face-to-face with his problem, his speech therapist, and other children who stutter in a joint attack on the bugaboo of stuttering. Therapy may be conducted individually or entirely in a homogeneous group composed of several youngsters. A combination of approaches, that is, group sessions interspersed with individual sessions as the need arises, is an ideal arrangement.

Active conscious avoidance of words and situations, though frequently encountered, is not necessarily habitual or consistent at this stage of development. Considerable variation is found among the children concerning the degree of word and situation anxiety. As the children progress through this stage of development, speech anxiety does become more acute. But most of the children talk without excessive reticence even in pressure situations. Fear* of

---

* The word *fear*, as used in this chapter, refers to anticipation of word difficulty (however low in consciousness) and to frustration (however slight) (4).

talking may be growing but is not necessarily well-established. Because such fears and avoidances are not well-established, attempts to build an objective attitude* need not be given emphasis in the therapy program for Phase Three stutterers. In fact, overemphasis on developing an objective attitude at this stage of development may create additional problems by focusing the child's attention on an accumulation of experiences that he may not have given too much thought to before. Fear may be a part of a child's experience but not perceived of yet as a necessary or consistent accompaniment of word and situation difficulty. Some children may indeed need help in reducing their fear of specific words and situations, but the reduction of fear is probably accomplished more easily and less dangerously by providing successful speaking situations than it is by direct discussions and strong urging to enter feared situations. This is not to say that efforts should not be made to encourage Phase Three stutterers to stutter openly without dodging or hiding their stuttering. On the contrary, we want them to eliminate their avoidance mechanisms before they do become strongly fixed. But this can be done without insisting that the stutterer accept a philosophy of "I am a stutterer and I intend to advertise this fact to everyone to whom I speak."

### Common Objectives for the Initial Therapy Period

Although the amount of emphasis will vary from child to child, the first stages of therapy should contain the following objectives:

Helping the child to understand the nature of therapy.
Helping him develop realistic personal goals for helping himself.
Helping the stutterer to be less sensitive about his stuttering.
Developing a healthy clinical relationship with the child.

Each of these is discussed in detail below.

---

* The objective attitude referred to here is part of a therapy approach that would encourage the child to admit to himself and others that he stutters but would rather not. Therapy approaches that utilize this concept often urge stutterers to "advertise" the fact that they have a problem. This type of approach is most useful for Phase Four stutterers—persons who have become thoroughly convinced that they are hopelessly handicapped and who have such habitual mechanisms of hiding their stuttering that any act of "disfluency" or any sign of "being different" is intolerable. In Chapter Six, more will be said about the application of the objective attitude to Phase Four stutterers.

*Helping the Child Understand the Nature of Therapy*
*and Helping Him Develop Realistic Goals for Therapy*

For those who work in therapy day after day, it is easy to forget that a child who comes in for speech help may not have the same perceptions or expectations about therapy as his therapist. It is the job of the therapist to structure the therapy situation in such a way that the child feels comfortable and secure and has a reasonable understanding of what will happen to him. Children frequently have misconceptions of therapy. Due to our modern emphasis on consulting those who seem to know best, whether it be the family doctor or dentist, a knowledgeable shoe salesman, or a Y.M.C.A. camp director, children and their parents expect to listen to appropriate suggestions and react to them as best they can. But for the most part, they are on the receiving end; the responsibility for what will happen is shouldered by the person they have gone to see. The same expectations are often encountered in the initial stages of speech therapy. One of our first tasks is to convince the child and, whenever possible his parents, that something will not be done *for* him, but *with* him. He will have an active role, not a passive one, and even though the responsibility for the success of therapy will be shared, he will have to shoulder a considerable portion of it. Unless he does so, therapy will not be very fruitful.

It is important too that the child set realistic goals for improvement. Often, due to the well-intended but misleading assurances of teachers and parents, the stuttering child expects his therapist to give him a few magical tricks which will relieve him of his stuttering blocks. Very early in discussions with the stutterer, it should be pointed out that therapy works toward *modifications* in attitudes and speaking behavior. It may be helpful to point out that speech habits become very well-established by frequent repetitions day after day, hour after hour, moment after moment. But, at the same time, overemphasizing the gradualness of speech improvement must not be permitted to create discouragement. Therefore, the child must be encouraged to accept short-term goals as rewards—he should be encouraged to see that any improvement is better than no improvement at all.

If he is under strong pressure to improve rapidly so that he can justify the time he spends in therapy, he must be provided with accomplishments to demonstrate at home, or ways of fending off these pressures. A basic understanding of the intent of therapy and the procedures to be followed in the therapy program will help him withstand these pressures better. Understanding is the key. If he knows what is going on, what is to come, and where he is in therapy, he will be much less anxious about himself and better able to cope with his parents or teachers if they expect too much from him too soon. It helps to give the stutterer some idea of the probable rate and type of progress he will make, to point out that many children attend regular therapy sessions for approximately a year or more and that they have frequent check-up visits after that. It should help him to know that a cure is not the usual result of therapy, but that he can expect, if he is growing more afraid to talk, fewer and fewer instances of being afraid to talk as therapy progresses. The therapist should make certain the child understands that he can learn to look better and sound better even as he stutters. In other words the aim is to specify the types of benefits he can reap from therapy and state them in terms he can understand.

## Helping the Child to Be Less Sensitive about His Stuttering

Unless the child is able to talk freely about himself and about his problem at this stage of development, therapy will be difficult, and the chances of relapse will be greater.

One way to decrease sensitivity about a problem is to learn more about it. "Learning more about it" means many things, but important among them is to learn what *it is not*. The child should know that it is not a matter of how bright or dull he is and it is not that something is basically wrong with him. Learning what *it is* means he should know what it is he *does*. He should know that he tenses up or strains on certain words, actively believing that he can't say them. But he *does* this. It doesn't just happen to him. He should know that he is a normal individual except for his stuttering and that stuttering is a problem that can be tolerated even by the possessor. We have found it helpful to use examples of famous persons who stutter—television stars, athletes, etc. We also like to mention other famous persons who have other types of handicaps—always keeping in mind that our task is to help the child feel less sensitive—less alone with his difference.

Sensitivity about stuttering can be decreased if the therapist always speaks of it calmly and matter-of-factly. If his behavior indicates to the child that he is not concerned about the act of stuttering and especially not ashamed of it (as a parent might be)—that he understands the nature of it—that he is not embarrassed by it, the child is likely to respond to these attitudes favorably. Such behavior does more than thousands of words about how one should not be sensitive.

Even though a child may be able to speak freely and frankly about stuttering, he should also be able to observe and tolerate specific examples of stuttering behavior—both his own and the stuttering (or pseudostuttering) of others. This is best done by the therapist asking questions about the type of stuttering exhibited by the child immediately following a stuttering block. These questions, stated calmly and objectively, should be aimed at helping the child notice specific aspects of his own stuttering behavior. For example, a therapist might find it relevant to inquire, "When you stuttered that time on your name, which sound did you seem to be having trouble on?" This can be followed up by other questions designed to focus attention on those aspects of the block which the therapist feels are most important, such as "Where did you seem to feel most tense?" "What were your lips doing on that block?" The child might be encouraged to repeat a stuttered word imitating the original as closely as possible and to notice specific aspects of his speech behavior. When a child is unable to imitate his own stuttering, he is generally very sensitive about it. This should prove a valuable index of the progress of therapy.

Another procedure which will help a child to learn to tolerate his own stuttering is to have him keep a record of the words on which he stutters so that he may compare this list with one kept by the therapist. Other assignments of a similar nature could involve having him count the stuttered words of other stutterers (instead of his own) and keeping a list of associated reactions used by himself or other stutterers.

Another way to decrease sensitivity—and one closely related to the ability to tolerate one's own stuttering behavior—is to learn to observe unemotionally and objectively the *reactions* of others to stuttering. Some children need to do more of this because they have encountered more scorn, pity, amusement, or other similar negative reactions. These children have encountered such negative reactions often enough to be on the defensive, and for very good reason. Some children can swallow large doses of this bitter medicine without ill effects. Some are so hypersensitive to what someone may think or feel that they imagine and conjure up hostile audience reactions when none exists. The stutterer has enough troubles without fighting straw men. If his audience is hostile, he should combat their hostility realistically. He must realize that if his listeners have a negative opinion of him, they will find confirmation in several outward signs. If they see signs that the child does not have a good opinion of himself, he has no right to expect them to hold him in high regard. His audience doesn't judge him entirely on the way he talks. They judge him on the way he stands, or the way he looks at the person he is talking to. If he slouches, averts his head, and avoids eye contact they can't help feeling that he is ashamed of himself. He signals too loudly. He shouts his feelings about himself even though he doesn't say it in words. High on the list of first things first is good eye contact. He may not be able to start out by controlling his stuttering, but he can control this particular feature of his behavior. Many clinicians attack this first because the child can do something concrete during an actual moment of stuttering. He can learn to do something of a positive nature for himself, independent of his stuttering, which will help pay dividends in improved self-confidence. He may see how long he can talk in front of a mirror before his eyes waver or look away or see if he can tell the color of the eyes of several people to whom he talks. Such practice may help him to know when he is making poor eye contact. If he can maintain eye contact and demonstrate poise even when he is having a severe block, he may find that some people will admire him for doing so.

## Developing a Healthy Clinical Relationship with the Child

The factors involved in building an appropriate relationship with a child are difficult to describe. Therapists who seem to have a knack for building good rapport are able to convey a sincere feeling that they accept the child as an interesting individual whom they would like to know better. They show a healthy interest in the child's stuttering and don't protest too much about his basic normality. They readily admit that his speech may be different, but they don't aggravate the problem by insisting that it really doesn't matter. Their manner indicates that they want to help as would any friend. But, as with friends, they have no intention of forcing their friendship. They show a nice appreciation of what it means to be in trouble. Successful therapists convey their respect for the child's individuality and his quandary.

Not all of these qualities and abilities come about instinctively. Therapists can learn ways to be helpful. For example, they can show in unobtrusive ways that they understand something of how a child feels as he stutters: "I'll bet it felt kind of scarey when you stood up there in front of the room to give that book report," or "It seems as if you know what you want to say, but sometimes the words get stuck and won't come out." Sometimes the therapists' questions reveal their knowledge of what stutterers do when they stutter; for example, "Do you ever switch to an easier word when you think you are going to get stuck?"

Unquestionably, rapport is a matter of being able to convey to the child that in the therapist he can find not only a source of understanding, a person who knows some answers to some rather pressing questions, but also a source of strength. Thus the successful therapist not only shows that he knows as much as he can know about stuttering, but he also shows that he can talk about it freely without ambiguity or reservations. He not only demonstrates that he can point out and discuss patterns of troublesome behavior, but that he believes in action and that he is willing to help the child do something constructive, and he is willing to do it now—the sooner the better. By precept he shows that stuttering doesn't frighten him. He can look at it without flinching and he is willing to stutter himself, any time, at the drop of a hat, without giving so much as a second thought to the consequences of having done so(7).

Once established, rapport isn't necessarily self-sustaining. How to start is important but what is done all through therapy is also important. Obviously, individual conferences permit the child to see that the therapist is interested just in him, but his understanding of the real intentions will be reinforced when he sees the same attitudes, empathy, and understanding shown to other children in a group. The child needs to know that the therapist is consistent in his beliefs and actions—that the attitudes expressed when talking about him are the same as when speaking to him.

The first stage of therapy, therefore, is concerned primarily with the development of a kind of relationship which will enable a child to benefit from therapy and will decrease his sensitivity about stuttering to the point where he will be able to begin to modify it. The objectives listed above can be stated in other ways or subdivided into many more goals, but, essentially, they exemplify the type of activities that will be necessary at the beginning of the therapy program. If these early stages of therapy are not given careful attention, considerable resistance is likely to be encountered when an attempt is made to move to later stages of therapy where so much more is demanded of the stutterer.

The remainder of this chapter is concerned with the core of stuttering therapy for the confirmed stutterer, that is, the displacement of maladaptive behavior, both overt and covert, during moments of communicative stress, by more adequate adaptive behavior. Although the discussion includes approaches to modification of the stuttering child's self-evaluational system, the main emphasis is concerned with approaches for the modification of characteristic nonproductive phonetic attacks on words.

### The Modification of Maladaptive Approaches to Difficult Words and Situations

A new set of goals and objectives must be kept in mind to help a child modify his maladaptive stuttering. Briefly stated, they are as follows:

> *Helping* him eliminate his unsatisfactory methods of approaching difficult words and situations.
> *Helping* him cope with and modify his struggles and postspasm reactions.
> *Helping* him cope with and displace his nonproductive anticipatory behavior with more adequate phonetic attacks on words.

Before plunging further into therapy methods and procedures, more explanation is offered of why and how a person who stutters continues to be confounded in his predicament. Only in this way can these therapy approaches make sense. This rationale for the modification of stuttering suggests that stuttering behavior becomes what it becomes, not because there is something inherently wrong physiologically or biochemically with the children who get into this kind of pickle, but because they see their own talking as difficult and unmanageable and reinforce this concept by making inferences, from their past experiences, which tend to impair fluent speech. This approach suggests that there is not necessarily something wrong "inside" a person to begin with.

In the preceding chapters it was pointed out that the stutterer "becomes" a stutterer because he eventually becomes convinced that reactions to his speaking are unfavorable—perhaps justifiably so because of what he was doing, that is, passing through stages of normal disfluency, encountering and reacting to emotional tensions of various sorts, or having difficulty learning to talk intelligibly. Members of the child's audience eventually observe a growing supply of evidence to help reinforce their own conclusions that his speech is abnormal and whenever enough of the right people are able to communicate their damaging appraisals effectively the circle is complete. Evidence of stuttering begets evidence of stuttering. The feedback of audience reaction now stimulates the stuttering response because the child has learned mostly wrong responses. These wrong responses can be exemplified by what a child does when he senses he will have trouble with a word.

When a child has stuttered long enough to learn to anticipate trouble with certain words and certain situations, he begins to develop a tendency to put off and avoid words and situations where there is a strong expectancy of stuttering. Some avoidance patterns are highly conscious—such as in the deliberate reply, "I don't know," to a question in which the stutterer sees a difficult word he will have to use if he answers the question correctly. Often, however, the avoidance patterns are almost subconscious. This is especially true of the quick retrials, postponements, revisions, and hesitations that the stutterer employs when he suddenly finds himself almost on top of a troublesome word.

To help a child eliminate his avoidance behaviors, it is important that he understands what it is that he must change and why it is reasonable that he should make these changes. The therapist also needs to remember that the things a child does when confronted with difficult words constitute his attempt, whether appropriate or inappropriate, to solve a problem under duress. When a child is confronted by a word that he suspects he may stutter on he tries to protect himself. His needs are several: he needs to feel fluent, he needs to get to the end of his sentence or thought, he needs to maintain the approval of his audience, etc. The behavior he chooses is limited to what is available to him. It is limited by what he has done in the past under similar circumstances, by his physical capabilities, by the pressures of the environment in which he lives, by what he has observed someone else do, or by what he has been taught to do. If he chooses the right behavior from among his available behaviors things go well for him. His momentary lapse may be soon forgotten. If he makes the wrong choice he may be able to recognize it as a wrong choice and try something else more appropriate next time. But, possibly in desperate straits, he may not have a previous favorable experience to fall back on. What does he do when there is no appropriate, prescribed behavior available? He improvises.

A child may learn to avoid certain words for similar reasons. Under the threat of an imminent breakdown in communication he realizes he must do something so he does what he does because he has to do something. To wait out the threat of a block or tremor to see if it will subside may likely be the behavior he first attempted early in his stuttering career, because one learns to do nothing, at least at first, in the face of danger. Doing nothing thus may turn out to be the smart thing to do because the tremor-inducing tension may subside. Or, if the tension doesn't subside, he may find it expedient to try another, easier word, to back up and try again, or to use any other rewarding behavior that will resolve his dilemma even if only temporarily. Once he finds a trick or device that will help him solve his dilemma this "crutch" will be called on again and again.

Some children find that these fortuitous expediencies suffice to get them out of their temporary difficulties and their confidence in speaking is not seriously affected. As their confidence in themselves rises for a variety of reasons and because their lack of ability to speak on occasions has not proved insurmountable, tensions and anxieties relating to these occasions now begin to subside and become infrequent occurrences. As the possibility of communication breakdown becomes more remote, maladaptive stuttering as a reaction to communication threats becomes an infrequently used and relatively impotent behavior reaction. Manifestations of stuttering in these children never gain a foothold and it is said of these children that they "outgrew" their stuttering.

Unfortunately, some children are not lucky enough to stumble on a fortunate combination of expediencies during early speaking crises. Even though they may use the same avoidance devices and tricks as do those children who eventually shed their stuttering behavior, circumstances differ—tensions and pressures come in all amounts and motivations vary. We all generalize about the similarity of circumstances and most of the time we can safely do so. But when a child who tends to view talking as difficult incorrectly judges the difficulty of a situation and especially when he underestimates how tense he is, the device or trick he calls on to help him through his crisis may not work. He tries to let the tension subside, but it doesn't subside; he backs up for a running start, but still the words appear impassable. His anxiety mounts and he may have to struggle with a word, but, this does not mean he will abandon the device. It has served a purpose before and in the emotional throes of his need to communicate he is not inclined to be analytical. Unless he rejects a particular behavior early he is likely to perseverate in this behavior simply because it is available to him. Where there are several behaviors to choose from, the better facilitated behavior is likely to be chosen first and thus maintains its dominance. In some situations with some words he may go through his entire repertory of available behaviors and even improvise new ones, but the facilitated behavior, which helps him just enough, will be maintained. The important thing to keep in mind is that avoidance behavior is facilitated because it meets a need. It staves off, no matter how ineffectively or temporarily, the terrors of the tension tremor.

In the later stages of stuttering—Phases Three and Four—the usual focus of attention in diagnosis and therapy is on feared words and situations and on the muscular tremor accompanying these stuttered words. By the time a child has progressed to Phase Three and without question by the time he has reached Phase Four, it is almost impossible to describe "stuttering" succinctly. Explanation is difficult because of the many and varied maladaptive adjustments children come up with as they attempt to "get over their stuttering." For one thing they view their trouble as a "block." Stutterers, even as young children, can be observed to "push" through their words, and as they get older they frequently refer to being "stuck." Any number of parts of our anatomy can get stuck if we think enough about the dreaded possibility. Most of our muscular systems respond to excess muscular innervation by "sticking." For example, if the great orbicularis oris muscle is innervated strongly enough, the lips will close tightly. If the breath stream is pushed violently against this barrier, tensions can be felt extending well into the abdominal region. If the "push" is increased, the lips can be made to tremble and if vocalization is attempted under these highly unfavorable circumstances, the results are catastrophic from a speaking standpoint. Not only are the lips, diaphragm, and vocal cords thus capable of sticking, but so, too, is the tongue. When the tongue is forced against the palate a tremor may radiate to the chin, tension may be felt and observed in the neck muscles and again the entire respiratory and phonatory system may be locked up in a manner inappropriate to speaking.

Critical here are the excessive tensions and inappropriate phonetic attempts that are brought into play when a word is considered difficult. Because the anticipation of difficulty by the stutterer conjures up "push," the proper conditions for "being stuck" are available. The tremor, which is the result of excessive muscular tension, is viewed by the possessor as evidence that something is happening to "cause" the trouble.

Of even more critical importance, however, is the fact that stuttering becomes self-perpetuating. During the approach-avoidance conflict period prior to the actual moment of crisis, muscular tensions are set up which beget stuttering. The ensuing struggle behavior, here equated with stuttering, is punishing and unpleasant. While in the throes of stuttering, the stutterer works desperately to stop it, and once he does so his anxieties and tensions subside. The sense of relief that comes with the cessation of the block reinforces the drive and much of the reason for absorbing the punishment, anxiety, and tension during the block, because the act of stuttering tends to dissipate the anxiety which had set up the crisis in the first place.* Thus emerges a pattern of stuttering composed of several parts:

---

* Several sources are available for the reader who wishes to read more about the reinforcement of stuttering symptoms.

Harold L. Luper, "Consistency of Stuttering in Relation to the Goal Gradient Hypothesis, *Journal of Speech and Hearing Disorders*, XXI (1956), 336-42.

Joseph G. Sheehan, "Theory and Treatment of Stuttering as an Approach-Avoidance Conflict," *Journal of Psychology*, XXXVI (1953), 27-49; and, "Conflict Theory of Stuttering," in J. Eisenson (ed), *Stuttering: A Symposium* (New York: Harper & Row, Publishers, 1958), pp. 125f.

Charles Van Riper, *Speech Correction: Principles and Methods*, Fourth Ed. (Englewood Cliffs, N.J.: Prentice-Hall, Inc., 1963) pp. 334f. Also by Van Riper:

(A) Anticipation of trouble
(B) Trouble (the moment of stuttering)
(C) Relief (the reduction of fear following an episode of trouble)

The problem encountered in the management of stuttering re-
volves around the question of where one effectively attacks this
well-integrated pattern of behavior. Seemingly at (A), for if the
expectancy of stuttering could be lowered or eliminated then the
tensions would not be encountered at (B), and part (C) would
not need to be considered. This approach does work well when
the child is in Phase One or Phase Two stuttering. The child
has not been thoroughly conditioned at these stages of development. He has not been sufficiently punished by ridicule, pity, or
rejection to enter into the strong approach-avoidance conflicts
which precipitate stuttering tremors. In Phases One and Two the
system can be prevented from becoming a well-integrated pattern
through active manipulation of a child's environment aimed at
decreasing the anxiety-inducing stimuli or the anticipation of
trouble. But in Phase Three, the child is already actively engaged
in trying to forestall trouble through the use of avoidance devices
and tricks. Because he has been conditioned to encounter trouble
and has experienced relief through the act of stuttering, provisions
for penalty-free talking during therapy sessions may possibly elicit
fluency *but only during therapy sessions.* In the give-and-take of
talking in a competitive, free-for-all situation, little carry-over, if
any, will be observed. Van Riper points out that a stutterer does
not solve his problem merely by experiencing a period of free
speech. He emphasizes that the effects of suggestion and situation
are temporary, and that that type of self-confidence is affected by
too many other factors to render it a permanent foundation for
fear-free speech (9:379).

By Phase Three systematic therapy is aimed at breaking up the
child's pattern of avoidance and the conditions that reinforce
the stuttering. Strong clinical demands are sometimes made on the

---

Chapter 27, "Symptomatic Therapy for Stuttering," in L. C. Travis (ed), *Handbook of Speech Pathology* (New York: Appleton-Century-Crofts, 1957).

George J. Wischner, "Stuttering Behavior and Learning: A Preliminary Theoretical Formulation," *Journal of Speech and Hearing Disorders,* XV (1950),
324-35.

An excellent summary statement of this point of view also can be found in
Oliver Bloodstein, *A Handbook on Stuttering for Professional Workers* (Chicago:
National Society for Crippled Children and Adults, Inc., 1959), pp. 58f.

child to eliminate his attempts to avoid or otherwise minimize his stuttering. Therapy is also aimed at the aspect of the stuttering that reinforces the stuttering—the relief the child experiences with the cessation of the stuttering. At times demands are placed on the child to let his stuttering come—he is not to repress it—he should stutter out in the open so that it can be observed, analyzed, and then modified.

Once the child is able to do something constructive *before* and *after* the block, therapy is aimed at modification of his struggle *during* the block. Finally, provisions are made to help him cope with his previously nonproductive anticipatory behavior and to replace this behavior with more adequate phonetic attacks on words. Means for helping a child to meet these demands of therapy will be discussed in detail.

### Helping the Child to Cope with His Approach-Avoidance Conflicts

In order to eliminate his avoidance behavior a child must be able to recognize it, reject it, and substitute in its place a readiness to stutter openly and freely without hiding, repressing, or disguising his stuttering.

In order to recognize his avoidance behavior, a checklist of various avoidance mechanisms should be prepared. Several devices which the child himself uses should be included in this list. He may carry this list with him to keep a record of the devices he observes as he pays attention to his speech in several different specific situations or in several short conversations during a therapy session. To keep the child from feeling he is being penalized, he himself should make most of the judgments concerning which secondary reactions he uses. In this way, not only is he kept from thinking that his every word is being watched for mistakes (which may be the very thing that made him anxious about his speech in the first place), but also he can learn to take responsibility for his own speech behavior—a necessity if he is to be at all successful in modifying his stuttering. Also, he should be encouraged to let his blocks come out in the open. If he is to repress anything he should repress his desire to keep from stuttering. The checklists may be changed slightly from day to day to focus attention on the different avoidance mechanisms he uses. As a rule, it is more helpful to call his attention at first to those mechanisms of which he is aware. After he is able to point out and do something about his more obvious avoidances, his attention can be directed to avoidances which are unconscious or which he tends to deny.

### Nonrecognition of Avoidance Devices

Some children use avoidance devices of which they seem to be completely oblivious—they may even deny their existence when the therapist points them out. When this happens, the therapist should look into the possibility that the child does not fully understand what is wanted of him. Perhaps the rationale justifying the elimination of these devices isn't convincing; more often, the instructions and directions aren't clear. The child may not understand how he should signal his recognition of avoidance. There are many ways, for example:

> He can say, "There's one," directly after whatever it is he wants to point out.
> He can repeat deliberately the same starter phrase a second or third time.
> He can make a tally of his "ums" or his "ers" or other devices.

Nonrecognition of avoidance devices may mean that this new way of solving his problem is too threatening to the child. Perhaps the child's fear of stuttering is so great that he cannot bring himself to make a direct attempt on a stuttered word. Perhaps the kind of relationship with the child which provides an immediate reward through simply being able to do what is asked of him has not been established. Perhaps there has not been judicious use of praise and encouragement. The possibility that stuttering is in some way serving as a reward for the child should also be considered. For example, stuttering may be rewarding if it brings a child the increased parental attention he thinks he needs. Stuttering may also have reward value if it serves as a "good excuse" for unsuccessful school performance. The child's resistance or apparent resistance should lead the therapist to examine several possibilities.

With some children, the use of increasingly specific questions along the lines suggested above is needed to help them see what they are doing. Sometimes it is necessary to have them listen to their own recorded speech so that specific devices can be acknowledged. It is extremely important though that the therapist refrain from forcing a child to admit or give up devices which he feels are helping him. The therapist should always realize that the child who clings to inappropriate behaviors has a reason for doing so. Greater efforts might be expended to explain and demonstrate the inappropriateness of avoidances, but excessive pressure and threat should not be used.

## Avoiding Avoidance

In order to modify a child's unsatisfactory manner of approaching difficult words and situations, the therapist should develop in him a willingness to talk in difficult situations and to use difficult words deliberately without avoidance. This is especially important for a person well along in Phase Three stuttering. His unsatisfactory approach to stuttering has previously consisted of various avoidance devices. To counteract this, he should be encouraged to feel "brave" or "courageous" about facing such difficult tasks. Some of this involves suggestion. The therapist shows that he recognizes that saying a highly dreaded word is a tough task— it is hard to do. And, whenever he sees even a little effort on the child's part to face a situation or to tackle a given word without avoidance, praise is given for such courage. The child knows that here is an adult who recognizes how difficult it was and who is proud of him. Immediate rewards are introduced for eliminating avoidances. The child is praised for what he is able to do, without being punished for those times when his courage falters. He becomes more willing to tackle anxiety-loaded situations just for the reward of "being brave." As he does more and more of this, the rewards tend to multiply because he finds the words easier to say.

When the child begins to feel the glow of his bravery, he should keep a list of the hard words he attempts without avoidance and the situations he has deliberately entered without procrastination. This provides another reward. This helps him to remember, as his fear of speaking situations decreases, how much improvement he has made in this respect.

Here is an illustration of one of several ways of discussing this critical aspect of stuttering with a youngster:

> Remember the first time you went off a high diving board? Supposing you went all of the way up to the top of the ladder and then instead of going out on the board you backed down. Your fear probably would be much greater the next time you tried to go up simply because you gave in to it before. Now you have to

worry not only about hurting yourself when you jump, but you have to worry about how much courage you have. Or, suppose you stood up there on the edge of the board and kept trying to get up the nerve to go off. Each time you hesitated you probably were more afraid than the times before. How did you finally do it? You just jumped right off. You made yourself go right ahead and do the thing you were afraid of doing. And if you kept right on— just going back up and jumping off—it became easier to do each time you did it. The same thing is true of stuttering. Whenever you come to a feared word or a feared situation, if you back off from it, or put off saying it, your fear will build up. Only when you can get yourself in the habit of going right ahead and making one strong attempt to say the word will your fear finally begin to decrease. But it won't disappear all of a sudden. You'll find, though, that as you eliminate your pussyfooting, your fear will let up.

This type of approach definitely smacks of suggestion and salesmanship but we make no apologies for it. We feel that the child needs quite a bit of encouragement to begin something that seems unnatural.

Other helpful approaches to aid the therapist in convincing the child of the importance of eliminating avoidances may be found in the workbook, *Self-Inventory* (5) by Chapman, and in Van Riper's *Speech Correction: Principles and Methods,* Fourth Edition (9).

This new pattern of adjustment may be resisted simply because it is new and unfacilitated. The maladaptive behavior at this stage of stuttering is rarely habitual or stereotyped, but since it has been used before its relative strength is much greater, and it tends to reward its use by a reduction of fear and anxiety. Avoidance behavior may thus be strong enough to appear even in moments of slight stress, such as in casual conversation. During any speaking of consequence the relatively old, tested, facilitated pathways to adjustment will be chosen more often than the untried, unproven, and unfacilitated ones.

Think for a moment how a child might react to a request that he give up his avoidance behavior. He might justifiably interpret this request as, "Stop using all the tricks you have been using successfully to make it easier to talk. Give up your tested formula for an untested experiment. Go ahead, make a fool of yourself. Let your stuttering come out in the open so it can be seen, ridiculed, or pitied."

Naturally, few children will be willing to do this unless they can be convinced that these avoidances, though temporarily helpful, actually make the total act of speaking over a long period more difficult. A good case needs to be built, therefore, to get a child to consent to give up his known, immediate rewards for delayed rewards of unproven value. Moreover, other substitute rewards must be provided immediately to shore up the insecurity that may have been induced by modifying or eliminating the child's tried, if not true, behavior.

## Direct Attempts to Modify Stuttering Patterns

Eliminating avoidance devices is actually a process of doing something about stuttering, but it may not satisfy the child's urge to come to grips with, and rid himself of, his stuttering. Successful stuttering therapy actually provides a means to permit an ongoing effort at general self-improvement. Although the therapist himself cannot rid the child of his stuttering, he can provide a vital, philosophical tool to facilitate self-improvement and permit the eventual elimination of stuttering. He can show the child the way to go about his self-remodeling.

If a stuttering child is asked to tell what happened immediately after he has stuttered for a sentence or two, the predictable answer is, "I stuttered." He may not be able to tell the specific words. And when asked, "How did you stutter?" he usually looks at the therapist as if to say, "If I knew, I wouldn't have done it!" Herein lies the main ingredient to success in therapy. If the therapist is skillful in directing his client's attention to *what* he did, *when* and *how,* he may not have to spend too much time explaining *why.* By that time the child himself will have the essential answers and can demonstrate his insight by being able to do something satisfying, constructive, ego-supporting, and specific—in contrast to his former feeling that he was in the grip of something intangible, unspeakable, uncontrollable, and irreversible about which he could do nothing.

One early and necessary aspect of stuttering therapy invariably hinges on the ability of the therapist to point to, and insist that the child notice, stuttering on certain words (not all words) and in some situations more than in others. Thus, the wheat is separated from the chaff. The problem becomes a specific one rather than a general one. Willful action is given precedence over wishful thinking. Voluntary control over appetites, urges, desires, hunches, and inclinations is a sign of maturity. Self-control signals self-growth. But, in order to learn self-control, one must identify and recognize what should be controlled, inhibited, repressed, or modified. Moreover, evidence must be forthcoming that something can be done. Nothing much can be done overnight. But much can be accomplished step by step, part by part.

*Loose Contacts*

When a child has learned to make frequent direct attacks on his feared words, the therapist can begin to suggest more successful ways of using his articulators. Instead of using increased tension and excessive pressure, the child may be shown how to perform the same articulatory movements with reduced pressure. These "reduced-tension" beginnings on difficult words have been called "loose contacts" by Van Riper (8). Emphasis on this concept of smoothness and relaxation is especially helpful for younger stutterers. They should be encouraged to practice "easy stuttering" and to stutter deliberately as they concentrate on keeping their articulators relaxed, as in the following illustration:

> Push your fist against the table very hard. Notice that when you push it hard enough, your entire hand or arm begins to tremble. Now push your hand against the table but without much tension. Try the same thing with your tongue as you say "top." First, push it hard, then try it with only about half that much tension. When you stutter, notice that you usually push your tongue against your mouth very hard. But you can make that sound without so much tension. In fact, it's much easier to say the word "top" if you are not pushing hard.

Other similar examples help the child to understand the concept of reduced or optimal tension as opposed to excess tension. If he can learn to approach his words directly with reduced tension in his lips, tongue, or vocal cords, there is an excellent chance that his speech will improve dramatically without further therapy. In fact, with some stutterers we have known, therapy was discontinued at this point with very good results. With almost all of them, we find that the ability to say feared words without avoidance and with reduced tension greatly reduces the overt stuttering pattern and eventually the amount of anticipated difficulty.

## Cancellations

One of the most fundamental all-purpose tools in stuttering therapy is the technique of cancellation developed by Van Riper. Essentially, this technique consists of having the child attempt a stuttered word again, following a short pause. Van Riper explains the value of this technique as follows:

> Ordinarily the conclusion of an act of stuttering produces a reduction of fear and an escape from frustration. . . . Even though he immediately falls into another blocking, he at least escapes from fixation on the word that he had dreaded. This momentary feeling of relief has reinforcement value. It keeps the symptoms at full strength.
>
> The *postspasm period* is most important in therapy. This is the Achilles' heel of the disorder. To attempt to alter or control the prestuttering period is too difficult because of the intense fear. To attempt to modify the stuttering *immediately* by working on it during its compulsive course is similarly onerous. But in the period immediately following the stuttering we have our most favorable point of therapeutic attack. If we can do something constructive at this time, we can prevent repression from doing its evil work. This postspasm period is the best time for clear-thinking analysis of the stuttering behavior, for contact with the self. If we can use the postspasm period to contrast the maladaptive symptoms which have just occurred with a more efficient, less destructive form of non-fluency, then we will have attacked the disorder in its most vulnerable spot. Finally, and of greatest importance, by inserting a deliberate, voluntary bit of discriminatory behavior at this moment, we prevent the symptoms from being reinforced by the feeling of relief. Before the stutterer is free to continue with the remainder of his utterance, he must still go through the process of cancellation. Only the cancellation sets him free from communicative frustration. Therefore it will be the cancellation that gets the greatest reinforcemen from this source (8:421-22).

Although the instruction to the child varies with circumstances, the general procedure is as follows:

1. Have the block. Go through it any old way, but *don't stop* until you get through the word.
2. Stop. (Time varies, depending on the child's morale.) Use this pause to allow your speech mechanism to "return to a state of rest." Figure out what is going on during the block. (The loci of tension, pressure, tongue position, etc.)
3. Say the word again. If you stutter, OK. (Better if you stutter in a

different way—or see if you can stutter deliberately in the very same way you did to begin with.)
4. Continue the sentence until you stutter again.

After a child has mastered this form of cancellation he should then learn to do as follows:

1. Have the block.
2. Stop. Figure out what is going on in the block, loci of tensions, what you are thinking, how calm or emotional you are, etc.
3. Say the word again but in a different way. Bounce; loosen up your tension. Try to slow down the tremor rate on the cancellation attempt.
4. Finish the sentence.

There are a number of useful ways in which cancellation can be employed. Of first order of importance is that a communication system can be worked out wherein the child signals to his therapist that he knows that he has just stuttered. This helps the child isolate the block from the rest of his fluency and disfluency and pins down the fact that his stuttering is a discrete behavior related to words. Listed below are some other ways cancellation can be used:

Cancellation provides a way of modifying reactions to stuttering and analyzing the specific behaviors which the stutterer employs. For example, he can note the amount of tension he felt and rate it on a scale of one to ten or he can work on maintaining good eye contact on the cancellation attempt.

Cancellation can be used as a form of negative practice. See if he can make the cancellation an exact duplicate of the original.

Cancellation can help foster a philosophy of doing something about failures.

Cancellation can encourage a variety of available behaviors instead of habitual or stereotyped behaviors.

*Cautions in the Use of Cancellations*

This is only one technique to be used with a battery of techniques. It is not a complete stuttering therapy in or by itself. A cancellation itself is abnormal, and the therapist should keep this in mind if he meets resistance in its application, especially if the child is requested to use it outside of the therapy setting. Since a stutterer can often say a word successfully immediately after stuttering (on the after-beat) with relatively little trouble, he should make sure there is a significant pause before the cancellation. The child should always stutter his way entirely through the word before pausing and cancelling. Because cancelling may become a trick, it should not be used indiscriminately. Unless the child goes all the way through the word before pausing and cancelling, the whole technique will merely become a postponement trick. Cancellation should be continued only to the point where the stutterer can learn other skills in handling his blocks.

Cancellation encourages an ongoing attempt into feared words and has its real value in preventing repression of stutterings and consequent relief-rewards. Further, it permits a systematic means of analyzing and modifying inappropriate reactions. It isn't necessary that all children learn the name for this practice of stopping, analyzing, and trying the word again. Some children, when they learn that the technique has a label, turn cancellation into a magical ritual. Again, the therapist must guard against indiscriminate use. Simple repeating without a significant pause is to be frowned upon.

The therapist should keep in mind the multipurpose use that can be made of this approach. It permits specificity rather than generalities. Daily use of this technique during the first stages of therapy helps the child know that he can do something about his stuttering. At least he will be able to put a checkrein on his helter-skelter, willy-nilly, ungovernable plunges into and out of word difficulty and anxiety.

### Modification of Malreactions to Excess Tension During and After Overt Stuttering

Specific work is also needed to help the majority of confirmed stutterers gain confidence in their ability to speak when they find themselves already in the throes of a stuttered word. Stutterers don't stutter all the time to all people. Often a child will remain relatively relaxed and express himself spontaneously, un-self-consciously until the first occurrence of a stuttered word. Then he tenses up and has relatively more trouble speaking fluently than before. A series of stuttered words may thus be triggered by this "first" occurrence. If a child can learn to react to these occurrences of stuttering without these automatic, inevitable increases in tension, the frequency of stuttering will decrease, his apprehension of "having another block" will be lessened, his need to anticipate and avoid feared words will be reduced, and consequently his total speaking behavior will become much more spontaneous and less hesitant. A child acquires a feeling of confidence when he realizes that even if he does stutter he will be able to do something about it. This kind of confidence is much more beneficial than the false confidence that some persons try to instil in a child by suggesting that there "is really nothing to worry about."

*Campaign for the Elimination or Significant Reduction of Behaviors Associated with Attempts to Complete Stuttered Words*

As a pattern of stuttering becomes fixed, habitual mannerisms are developed which the child feels will help "release" him from the stuttering block. These particular devices develop from the child's belief that he is "caught" in the throes of his attempt to say the word—that he has no real control over what happens once he begins to stutter. The child may try to complete the stuttered word by forcing harder—by making his articulatory efforts more intense. As part of this forcing behavior, the child may screw up his face, make sudden jerking movements with his head, blink his eyes, raise the pitch of his voice, switch suddenly to an inhalation, or any number of other complicated attempts to struggle free from his excess tension. These forcings add to the picture of abnormality and make the task of completing the word more difficult. Again, as with the approach-avoidance devices employed by the stutterer to cope with a feared word, some of these behaviors are much more under voluntary control than others. Some are used quite consciously by the stutterer in the belief that they will enable him to "escape" from the block. Others are simply the result of the excess tension employed by the stutterer and are not at a very high level of awareness. For example, the increased rate of blinking and squinting that are seen in many stutterers when they force strongly on a word are usually quite unconscious. In fact, blinking rate is used in many psychological studies as a measure of tension and anxiety. Most of the abnormal breathing patterns seen in stutterers are also largely unconscious.

To begin to modify these unsatisfactory ways of stuttering, the stutterer should understand the nature of these behaviors and the necessity for eliminating or modifying them. Here again checklists are helpful especially if several different types of forcing behaviors are listed. The child may be asked to find examples in his own speech of the specific devices he commonly employs and to recognize these mechanisms in the speech of others as well as in his own speech.

With many stutterers it is easier to modify these inappropriate reactions if the first attempts at modification are made after the completion of the stuttered word. The cancellation technique is of special value here. During the pause after the block the child should analyze his tensions to determine where they were and what parts were fixed or locked. He should observe particularly whether he tried to move to the remaining part of the word. Many stutterers know their phonics when it comes to beginning sounds— few can readily tell the end sounds of feared words. The child could be asked to check whether he "shifted into neutral," that is, whether he let his tensed tongue or abdomen relax during the pause and to see whether he persisted in the same tensions as he tried the cancellations or words farther along in the sentence. By contrast, some children fail to start the word with the sound it begins with and some even attempt a word with no sound at all. These children need to realize this in order to attempt a more appropriate approach during the cancellation.

## Pull-Outs

When the child has become proficient in his ability to cancel and cancels the vast majority of his blocks satisfactorily under difficult circumstances, a shift can be made to a direct alteration of the block during its occurrence. Instead of letting the block run its original course, the child is now encouraged to modify the block before it is released so that it is released under control. This technique permits the same analysis and insights as in cancellation, but they now take place during the block itself. Essentially a pull-out is a way of gaining release from a block, but in a controlled manner. Instead of jerking and thrashing blindly, the child is encouraged to keep the block going voluntarily until he feels he can pull out of it at any time he wishes. If a blackberry vine hooks your clothing, you may get snagged tightly, skin and clothes, if you try to jerk free. There is little real danger to be found in a blackberry patch if you proceed carefully, but you may be in for some real trouble if you panic. Whether entangled in a blackberry patch or in a stuttering block, the only danger comes through losing your head. The child must be encouraged to stop his urge to forge ahead in his block unwisely. He should be encouraged to maintain the block until he knows he can pull out of it when he wants to, unhurriedly and smoothly. The child should be shown how he can throw himself into "real blocks," * maintain the duration of the block until he can accomplish what needs to be accomplished, then pull out smoothly. Directions may be given similar to these:

> Now that you can cancel successfully, you may have noticed that as you finish some of your blocks you try to jerk out of the tremor. Sometimes, even though you have completed the word you jerked back into the block. Your job now is to see if you can slow down those tremors while moving smoothly into the rest of the word. Remember, your pull-outs must be absolutely controlled, slow (at least at first) and you must have a loose, smooth, but strong movement as you move to the rest of the word.

Via pull-outs a child can learn that release from struggle behavior can be accomplished through a gradual relaxation of his tensed articulators or accomplished through shifting from a fixation or prolongation of the troublesome sound to a deliberate movement into and through the rest of the word. Instead of jerking out of a rapidly oscillating tremor, the child can learn how these rapid oscillations can be kept going, maintained longer than usual, and slowed down until there is no danger of being snapped back into the tremor again during the pull-out as would be the case if the tremor-maintaining tension was kept at its original high level. Ordinarily a child who gets out of a high-tension tremor successfully, that is, without being jerked back into it, does so by luck—he manages to make his shift into the word in phase with the tremor. In some tremors, the recoil back into the word occurs after the word is completed. This happens when the child increases the tension too much in order to move into the rest of the word, and when the shift is made out of phase with the tremor.

Part of the child's perseveration in a stuttered word is due to his attempt to make the word sound right. He must learn to know that once part of the word has been slurred or prolonged, once a syllable or sound has been repeated, the word is damaged

---

* A stutterer usually indicates that in a faked block, one which he enters into voluntarily, he knows that he can terminate it at any moment. A faked block changes to a real block, accordingly, when he is unsure of being able to finish the block at the exact moment he wants to.

beyond repair. The word will never sound right. The only thing he can do is to continue through the word with at least a modicum of grace. A normal speaker who trips on a word usually disentangles himself and says the word again. If he is ruffled by his mistake he may smile ruefully, but invariably he carefully says the word again to maintain intelligibility. A broken word is broken and cannot be repaired. To get disentangled with some kind of grace requires that an attempt be made to move on out to the end of the word with a semblance of self-control. One of the most vaunted virtues of the entertainment world is expressed in the words "The show must go on." Audiences appreciate the fact that the performer is operating under adverse conditions and tensions. Virtue lies in the attempt to do the best job that can be done under the circumstances. Loose contacts, cancellations, and pull-outs give the stuttering child the opportunity to show that he is willing and able to do something about the way he talks. Even though he is working under adverse conditions he can be relied upon to keep trying.

## Some Suggested Approaches for Using Pull-Outs

Have the stutterer practice stuttering voluntarily in different ways during the cancellation—increase tension, bounce, force, struggle, continue the block beyond its normal duration, etc.

As preparation for smooth pull outs have the stutterer (using real or faked blocks) try the following approaches:

> Throw himself into a real block.
> Maintain a real block until he is in control and the stuttering activity is all faked.
> Voluntarily shift the locus of tension from one part of the body to another during block.
> Try to release from block with sudden surge of tension.
> Try to maintain some other voluntary activity during block (finger tap, eye blink, movement of foot from side to side, etc.)

## Cautions Concerning Pull-Outs

The child must know when his moments of stuttering occur. He must be able to cancel satisfactorily 75 per cent or more of his blocks at any given time before beginning work on pull-outs. Strong demands for *smooth* transitions from the block to the rest of the word are often made. Jerking out of the tremor is not desirable. Tremors must be slowed down before attempting the transitions. In order to achieve this, the block may have to be maintained well beyond its normal duration. By the time the child attempts work on pull-outs, he must be reasonably able to avoid his avoidances and he must be able to attack the vast majority of his feared words directly and consciously. He should be able to throw himself into blocks, real or faked, without unreasonable qualms that the block itself might hurt him, be punishing, or make his stuttering worse.

## Phonetic Principles

Simple instructions to relax specific tensions and to keep moving through the word help make speaking easier for a child much more than do detailed descriptions concerning how to produce each sound of the English language. But there may be times when a child consistently has difficulty on certain sounds and where it is fairly obvious that he is using inappropriate methods either to get set for a word or to release his tension when in trouble. Some phonetic approaches are listed to suggest the kinds of things with which the clinician can help.

## Lip Sounds( P, B, M )

Obviously these sounds need to be started with the lips together. However, when a child attempts the sound with his lips pressed tightly together he will never be able to make the sound until he remembers the rest of the word, releases his lips, and moves into the rest of the word. He may be shown that he will never be able to say *baby* if he keeps his lips tightly shut. To say the word he must move to the next vowel. He may try to begin the word by saying "buh-buh-buh," even though the vowel is a long "a," not a schwa. It may help to say several lip-sound words to him, *boy, mama, paper, biscuit, peanut, mosquito,* and to have him tell you what vowel follows the initial sound.

## H

This sound causes a great deal of trouble because of the way it is normally produced. Phonetically it is the whispered form of the vowel that follows it. For example, the word *he* is produced as a voiceless *e* followed by a phonated *e*. The whispered part changes with the first vowel in the word. Some children feel all their breath slipping away on a word beginning with *h* because they feel that they have to say something out loud to say *h*. Actually if they understand the importance of slighting the *h* part and concentrating on the voiced vowel they would not so often have to find a substitute word for *hello* and *hi*.

## I

This speech sound is a word when said alone and refers to the person who is doing the speaking. But it is not a single sound. It is a diphthong made up of two parts resembling "ah" and "ee." It is critical here that the first part of this sound be started with voicing. The vocal cords should be making the *ah* noise, followed by a smooth transition into the *ee* part of the word.

## W and Y

These sounds illustrate the necessity for movement in talking. To say *we* it is necessary to start the word with a sound similar to long *oo* and move smoothly to *e*. The transition from *oo* to *e* provides the sound we recognize as *w* in the word *we*. Interestingly enough there is no *double-u* in *w*. All words starting with *w* start with a sound like *oo* but the vowel that follows may change. Nor is there a *why* in *y*. *Y* words start with a sound similar to *e* and the transition from *e* to the first vowel in the word provides the necessary sound. For example, to say *you* we say *e* then *oo*. To say *yellow* we only have to say the letter names of *E-L-O*, quickly, with smooth transitions to come up with the word *yellow*.

## Release Mechanisms

If a child uses release mechanisms which resist elimination, it is necessary to employ a more systematic plan for helping him eliminate this behavior. In these instances, the patterns of tensing and forcing which persist are reinforced so strongly that the speaker seems unable to prevent their occurrence. It is wise to ask the stutterer first to make *gradual modifications* of the behavior. For example, if his usual tendency is to throw his head backward when stuttering, begin by asking him to delay this tendency for a brief period. Slight modifications seem to be much easier to accomplish and often make it possible for him to make more drastic changes later. After several successful instances of using slight modifications of the characteristic behavior, he may modify the behavior more drastically—perhaps by using the same basic movement but in the opposite direction. For example, if a child jerks his head up when trying to release himself, he might be asked to lower it at the first impulse to raise it while watching himself in a mirror. The stutterer can usually make this type of modification. Perhaps it is because he feels the need for an accessory movement and any such movement will serve the same purpose. This type of contrast-modification has two advantages: (a) the deliberate modification of the stereotyped movement seems to weaken the strength of the habit, and (b) this type of deliberate modification brings the behavior up to a more conscious level of awareness.

If the behavior persists, some type of penalty can be arranged to increase his awareness of the behavior and to reduce its reinforcing properties. The penalties are not to be considered as punishments. More properly they should be of the nature of "reminding devices" such as the old trick of tying a string around one's finger. The penalty may take the form of an exaggerated negative practice where the behavior is deliberately repeated. The penalty may be a humorous act which the stutterer must perform before completing his utterance. Care should be taken to avoid embarrassing the child unduly or providing a secondary reward for the use of the behavior.

In summary, this phase of the treatment program consists largely of helping the stutterer change his habitual ways of reacting to the occurrence of stuttering. It involves both a change in his attitudes about the "dangers" concerning actual stuttering moments and a change in his speaking habits when stuttering is encountered.

### Reducing Specific Word and Situation Fears

Considerable reduction in word or situation fears will occur as a result of the previously discussed stages of therapy. But some stutterers, especially those in the advanced stages of Phase Three, greatly fear certain situations and words. Specific words and situations which are then anticipated with considerable anxiety will turn up as therapy progresses and should be kept in mind.

One of the first steps in reducing the fear of certain words or situations is to encourage the stutterer to verbalize why he is anxious about them. Frequently, a child will be unable to explain reasonably and objectively why he is so concerned. Bloodstein (2) has summarized a number of the findings concerned with conditions affecting the reduction or remission of stuttering and has arrived at the following generalizations about these conditions:

1. Stuttering varies with the degree of communicative responsibility felt by the stutterer.
2. Stuttering varies with the listener's reactions to stuttering, or with what they are imagined to be.
3. Stuttering varies with the need to make a favorable impression.
4. Stuttering varies with the amount, intensity, or the nature of "distractions" inherent in the speaking situations.
5. Stuttering varies in response to suggestion.
6. Stuttering varies with changes in physical tension.
7. Stuttering varies with the length of time elapsing between the moment the stutterer knows he is going to speak and his actual speech attempt.
8. Stuttering varies with the presence or absence of the cues to which it has become attached.

These findings can be related to the child's specific anxieties. It may help him to describe, confess, discuss, or specify what it is he fears. To pinpoint his anxieties may help him to understand why his fears came about in the first place.

### Campaign for the Reduction of Fear

After the child displays a reasonable understanding of the nature of the development of fears, his difficult situations or words can be analyzed to see what is difficult about them. Perhaps he consistently employs some form of behavior which makes speaking more difficult. Perhaps there is some reason (other than speech) why he tenses up in a particular situation. One stutterer we knew was very anxious about giving oral reports to his class. He even refused to go to school some days when he knew he would have to give a report. When he was taught more effective means of organizing and presenting oral reports, his fears began to abate. Although his fear did not disappear completely, he was able to keep up his oral report assignments. In this instance, the acquisition of skill in preparing a report helped to reduce the fear of stuttering.

Probably one of the most important ways to reduce specific fears is to help the child develop a willingness to carry out a campaign for the reduction and eventual elimination of fear. The child will want to reduce his fear. When he understands the nature of his fear he will be in a good position to help himself overcome it.

The fear of words or situations may be reduced by the principles of conditioning—in this instance the fear is to be extinguished. The goal is to provide the occurrence of the anxiety-producing event but without the accompanying negative reinforcement.

The therapist should help the child plan a series of steps of gradually increasing difficulty. For example, the child could either read or give an extemporaneous report to one individual, then to two or three, then to a larger group. Finally he should be willing to present his report to his class. The campaign for the elimination of fear should include repeated use of the feared word and repeated entries into the feared situation. It is the therapist's responsibility to ensure that these are successful situations for the child. Unless these situations provide some measure of success, the fear will probably not decrease. An important way to provide a feeling of success in feared situations is to encourage the child to focus his attention on some goal other than complete fluency. His new goal may be to try to get through all his blocks without becoming too flustered or simply to communicate effectively—with or without stuttering. The therapist can help the child devise many ways of concentrating upon aspects of speech other than fluency which can be rewarded.

The child should be encouraged to "cancel" by deliberately re-entering situations in which he feels he has failed. He should be encouraged to develop a basic attitude of willingness to go out of his way to re-enter situations in which he feels he has done poorly.

For specific feared words, the adaptation effect can be used to reduce stuttering. A particular feared word may be repeated over and over, keeping in mind that to practice a word out of context does not always involve the same tension and apprehensions as when the word is used in an actual speaking situation. Such practice should be aimed merely at reducing fear of the word to the point where the child is willing to attempt the word in a more critical setting.

### Developing New Speech Attitudes

The stutterer's problem does not end simply with the reduction of his fears and the attainment of less abnormal ways of speaking.

He must go still another step farther. The stutterer must learn to enjoy speaking—to enjoy it even more than most so-called normal speakers do. The speech therapist can do a great deal to foster the enjoyment of talking.

One way to develop a positive feeling about speaking is to help the stutterer place the optimum degree of importance upon "speaking correctly." Stutterers tend to exaggerate the importance of speaking properly and fluently. Barbara (1) feels that this is one of the dominant features in the development of stuttering. He calls it the *Demosthenes complex* and refers to the story of how the great orator overcame his handicap. As a child Demosthenes was weak and sickly. His movements were awkward, his voice weak, and because of a decided lisp his articulation was defective. In order to cure himself of the habit of shrugging up one shoulder, Demosthenes practiced speaking beneath a suspended sword that nicked his offending shoulder when he moved. To gain presence of mind in the face of the tumult, he matched his voice against the waves of the sea, and to cure his speech impediment he spoke with pebbles in his mouth. It was said that his sources of power as an orator were three—lofty morality, intellectual superiority, and the magical power of his language. Barbara goes on to say that people who have difficulty in speaking situations have a tendency to create an "image of Demosthenes." These people feel that if they could only speak clearly and lucidly at all times, they could conquer the world. They may imagine themselves specifically as great orators, holding vast audiences spellbound. Their speech begins to dominate their life activities to the exclusion of everything else, and compulsively they feel driven to excel in something which they feel is most lacking in themselves (1:101).

Stuttering tends to increase in those situations where the stutterer considers it important to speak perfectly. The feeling that speech is the most important part of one's life and that to speak perfectly is the only acceptable way to speak not only increases the stutterer's tension but takes away much of his enjoyment of talking.

Through examples from his own speech the therapist can demonstrate that "bobbles" in speech are not necessarily *important* blunders. He can give the stutterer assignments to count the disfluencies that occur in the speech of his teachers, his friends, or his favorite television stars. It may be pointed out that speech is only one small aspect of a person's total personality—only one of many parts reacted to by others. The acquisition of a new, positive approach to speaking depends on more than a rational discussion of the benefits of such an attitude; successful experience must reinforce the enjoyment of talking. The therapist can provide many emotionally satisfying, enjoyable speaking situations during the therapy sessions. He can include informal conversations about the child's interest, feelings about his teachers (positive or negative), discussions of his hopes and desires. The teacher's aid can be enlisted in providing a variety of enjoyable speaking situations outside of the therapy sessions.

Some parents actually do not know how to enjoy talking with their children. These parents find it helpful to sit in with their child during a therapy session to see firsthand how it is possible for an adult to enjoy talking with a child. What the parents really need to know is how to listen to their children. A good listener is the ingredient that makes for a good conversation. Johnson (6), in helping parents help their children overcome their stuttering, says, "The one thing you can do that will go farthest, in my judgment, to ensure that your child will grow up to be the clear-eyed, considerate, constructive person you want him to become is to teach him to be a good listener." Immediately he goes on to say that the way to do this is by being a good listener yourself.

> You wonder sometimes why he would ever say the things he does, but the point is you do wonder about it. You don't shush him. Maybe he's imagining things, some pretty fantastic things, but imagination is a wonderful, wonderful gift that flourishes with use —and just a little careful questioning now and then. Or maybe he's trying to tell you that he feels put upon, irritated, and outraged, and if you listen closely enough you might find out what his reasons are, and then you can do something about them if they seem important, or something about his way of looking at them if they don't(6:165).

### Modifying Other Factors Which Tend to Increase Tensions Associated with Speaking

We have been discussing modification procedures for the confirmed stutterer as if all of the child's anxiety and tension when speaking was the result of unpleasant experiences related to his stuttering. Although we do feel that a child who has stuttered for some time and whose stuttering patterns are relatively fixed perpetuates his problems by such tensions, other conditions can increase a child's anxiety about speaking. It is important, therefore, to seek out and reduce all possible areas of frustrating tension which may decrease a child's chances of speaking unconcernedly without undue self-consciousness or anxiety.

Speech centered conflicts will create tension in speaking. One of the authors recalls a child with a cleft-palate condition who began to stutter after he started school. It is difficult to speak properly with a cleft in the palate. In describing the development of his stuttering his mother indicated that she was unaware of any stuttering until her child had had several experiences at school where he was unable to make himself understood. There is good reason to believe that his embarrassment and his increased tension as he unsuccessfully tried to make himself understood led to his stuttering. Obviously, if a child has speech or language problems which make it difficult for him to communicate, these problems should receive prompt attention.

Conditions at home may contribute to a child's tensions. The storied simple life is mostly story. He may be teased by his sister, threatened by the impending arrival of a new baby, bewildered by moving from one city to another, anxious because his brother broke his arm, feel left out of things because he isn't old enough to join the Boy Scouts. It may be that perfectionistic attitudes and expectations on the part of his parents contribute to his tensions. If so, environmental therapy, such as discussed in Chapter Three, is indicated.

Since speech is our main avenue for relating with others, it is natural that interpersonal conflicts create tension which may result in stuttering. Any serious interpersonal conflict may increase the stutterer's over-all tension. If the therapist is trained adequately in dealing with emotional problems, he may approach these himself. In most instances, however, the child with an emotional problem that is not closely related to conditioned learning experiences of the stuttering should be treated by a qualified clinical psychologist or psychiatrist.

### Summary

This chapter describes a direct therapy approach for the modification of the speech symptoms of the confirmed (Phase Three) stutterer. Therapy measures include the modification of the child's unsatisfactory ways of reacting to his stutterings, reducing word and situation difficulties, providing for phonetic attacks on words, and developing new attitudes toward speech and speaking.

*References*

1. BARBARA, D. *Stuttering: A Psychodynamic Approach to Its Understanding and Treatment* (New York: The Julian Press, Inc., 1954).
2. BLOODSTEIN, O. *A Handbook on Stuttering for Professional Workers* (Chicago: National Society for Crippled Children and Adults, Inc. 1959).
3. ———. "The Development of Stuttering: II—Developmental Phases," *Journal of Speech and Hearing Disorders*, XXV (1960), 366-76.
4. ———. "The Development of Stuttering: III—Theoretical and Clinical Implications," *Journal of Speech and Hearing Disorders*, XXVI (1961), 67-82.
5. CHAPMAN, M. *Self-Inventory: Group Therapy for Those Who Stutter,* Third Ed. (Minneapolis: Burgess Publishing Co., 1959).
6. JOHNSON, W. *Stuttering and What You Can Do About It* (Minneapolis: University of Minnesota Press, 1961).
7. MULDER, R. L. "The Student of Stuttering as a Stutterer," *Journal of Speech and Hearing Disorders,* XXVI (1961), 178-79.
8. VAN RIPER, C. *Speech Correction: Principles and Methods,* Third Ed. (Englewood Cliffs, N.J.: Prentice-Hall, Inc., 1954).
9. ———. *Speech Correction: Principles and Methods,* Fourth Ed. (Englewood Cliffs, N.J.: Prentice-Hall, Inc., 1963).

# Chapter Six

## The Modification of Advanced
## Stuttering (Phase Four)

*At this advanced stage of development the possessor has vivid and continual anticipation of his stuttering, and it is viewed by him as a serious personal problem. Symptomatology is fully developed and is characterized by avoidance, postponement, starting, and release devices. Special difficulty is encountered in response to various sounds, words, situations, and listeners. The stutterer reacts emotionally to his stuttering. Fear and embarrassment are definite concomitants of his speaking problem. A child may be in high school before he reaches this level of stuttering, but all the features of Phase Four stuttering may be found in children as young as ten years of age. Cancellation, pull-outs, and loose contact techniques are employed as therapy approaches, but attention must now of necessity be directed toward the modification of malattitudes.*

In this last most advanced phase of stuttering, the child is deeply aware of his stuttering and tries his utmost to keep from stuttering. He may be quite artful in his attempts to hide or minimize his problem; usually, however, his avoidance attempts merely add to the bizarre abnormality of his problem. Avoidances of words and situations are now a habitual part of his speech behavior. Such avoidance is also a significant indicator of the seriousness of his distrust in his own ability to communicate.

The final back-breaking straw has been piled on the child who reaches Phase Four stuttering, and his previous, almost unconscious, suspicion about his speaking difficulty has now given way to a demoralized acceptance of himself as a person who has to struggle desperately just for survival as a talker. The Phase Four stutterer is acutely aware of himself, his stuttering, and the effect of his stuttering on his listeners. Since he now actively avoids both words and situations where unpleasantness is anticipated, attention must be paid in therapy to the emotions aroused by his anticipation of stuttering and the act of stuttering. Indeed, the emotional attitude of the speaker may be such that he finds it difficult, if not impossible, to discuss his stuttering openly and intelligently. To him, stuttering is an unmanageable affliction, a source of shame, an unspeakable stigma. Some stutterers at this phase are close to complete demoralization and are uncertain even of their inherent courage or strength of character. Having heard the frequent truism that "anyone can do anything if he only tries hard enough," and having failed countless times in his attempts to rid himself of the problem of stuttering, the stutterer may begin to feel that he lacks "will power." Phase Four stutterers often develop such strong sensitivities about their speech problem that they are unable to talk about it—even to themselves. Fully developed fear is now an active ingredient of talking and sensitivity about the problem of stuttering casts its shadow over almost everything the stutterer does.

### Encouraging the Desired Response

When children are so embarrassed about their speech problem that they cannot even talk or think about it unemotionally, it is difficult to get them to do what is necessary to overcome the problem. Their sensitivity about stuttering not only increases the handicapping effect of the stuttering but blocks any attempts to alter it. Dollard and Miller, after listing the basic steps in learning as consisting of drive, cue, response, and reinforcement, point out:

> Before any given response to a specific cue can be rewarded and learned, this response must occur. A good part of the trick of animal training, clinical therapy, and school teaching is to arrange the situation so that the learner will somehow make the first correct response. A bashful boy at his first dance cannot begin to learn either that girls will not bite him or how to make the correct dance step until he begins responding by trying(2:35).

And, to paraphrase Dollard and Miller, an embarrassed stutterer cannot begin to learn that stuttering can be tolerated or how to decrease the severity of his blocks until he begins responding by trying. One of the primary tasks of the therapist at this stage of therapy is to encourage the stutterer to face his problem long enough for new responses to occur and be reinforced.

The therapist should recognize that the Phase Four stutterer has greater difficulty in viewing his problem objectively than do stutterers at the other stages of development. He has generally stuttered longer, has experienced more failures, and has felt more frustrations. Often he has convinced himself that he is really different from other people. The world to him, is divided into two groups: the stutterers and the nonstutterers. All other differences become unimportant. The therapist when working with such a person may be puzzled to see the child refuse to carry out suggested assignments or refrain from attempts to talk in "easier, more normal" ways of talking. Some therapists may even suspect that the stutterer prefers to continue stuttering. Such is not often the case. The stutterer rarely wishes to continue stuttering, but neither does he feel he can keep from stuttering. Since he hates to admit his problem even to himself, and since his avoidance behaviors are well learned, he finds it difficult and even impossible to say his troublesome words in other ways.

In order to help the stutterer help himself, it is necessary that he reduce his sensitivity and embarrassment to the point where he can tolerate this deficiency in himself without undue anxiety. If his confidence has been shaken too severely, he may need supportive therapy for some time before attempting the more active parts of speech therapy. Some stutterers will require deeper psychotherapy before being able to work on their problem. But sooner or later the stutterer needs to face his problem differently. He needs to develop an objective attitude toward his problem to replace his defensive, emotional, subjective thinking about himself and the way he talks.

## The Objective Attitude

Van Riper (5) refers to the objective attitude as the intelligent, unemotional acceptance of an objectional difference as a problem capable of solution. This attitude is entirely different from the typical attitude of the Phase Four stutterer. This attitudinal change is not easy to accomplish, nor is a complete reversal in attitude a realistic goal here. Complete objectivity about one's self is seldom if ever achieved and it is not our purpose to suggest that this is a necessary or even desirable kind of behavior to aim for. The problem is this. The stutterer's attitude is usually charged with so much emotion and embarrassment that if he is ever to help himself he must first begin to change his thinking about himself. He needs to become *more* accepting and *less* emotional about what he does. This change in attitude does not require that he say, "I am a stutterer." But he does need to accept responsibility for what he does and is doing. In fact it may help to reinforce his so-called emotional, unintelligent behavior if he is taught to be "realistic" about himself and if he is encouraged to face up to his stuttering and to call himself a stutterer.

Objectivity, like honesty or faithfulness or other similar abstract concepts, involves both a way of thinking and a set of actions. The way of thinking, that is, the attitude, leads to certain desirable actions. The particular aspects of the objective attitude which need to be taught are those which lead to the actions considered to be desirable. Since the problems of the Phase Four stutterer are complicated so greatly by his habitual avoidance behaviors, the points stressed most in teaching the objective attitude are those which encourage actions opposite to avoidance. Below is a list of some of the specific attitudinal changes sought when teaching the objective attitude. They are not mutually exclusive.

1. The individual should feel a responsibility for his own behavior and for carrying out the changes that need to be made.

2. He should be willing, temporarily, to place greater emphasis upon how he talks and upon how he feels about speaking than on what he says.
3. He should be willing to allow others to know he stutters and should resist the temptation to hide or minimize his stuttering.
4. He should be willing to experiment with different methods for alleviating the severity of his problem.
5. He should desire to learn as much about the problem of stuttering as he can and about his own speech problem in particular.
6. He should become willing to enter difficult speaking situations even though he expects to stutter.

These aspects of the objective attitude are vital for the successful solution of the advanced stutterer's problem. It has been our experience that the major battle is fought here. If an objective attitude cannot be taught, the remainder of the therapy program may be fruitless.

## Assumption of Responsibility

At Phase Four, more than at any other stage of stuttering development, the success of therapy depends on whether the child assumes responsibility for his own behavior. When stuttering first starts, the responsibility for a change rests not on the child, but on his parents, his therapist, or any others who can change the conditions which precipitate an unusual amount of disfluency. As the child grows older and the stuttering becomes chronic, the perpetuation of the stuttering is in a large part self-initiated. A continually growing fear of stuttering and consequent attempts to avoid anticipated stuttering keep the stuttering going. Because the child now actively anticipates stuttering he now conscientiously attempts to keep from stuttering. He keeps his stuttering "hot" because of what he does to keep from stuttering. When he successfully avoids stuttering he maintains his dread of actual stuttering by assuring himself either consciously or unconsciously that his vigilance prevented the dreaded occurrence from taking place. When he does openly stutter he finds verification for the necessity of his vigilance. Avoidance helps to maintain his stuttering and his stuttering helps to maintain his avoidance. This circle must be broken. The success of therapy hinges on the child's willingness or readiness to break this circle. He must be able to stand up to his stutterings, to do something besides running and dodging from them. When he stutters or anticipates trouble he must be able to resist panic and experiment with and try out several new modes of behavior instead of giving in to his urge to duck anticipated unpleasantness, or to struggle to free himself from his blocks when in the throes of his trouble. He must be willing to try something different, but *he* must do it. He can be shown what to do, but the doing must be done by the child himself. Neither his therapist, his parents, nor anyone else for that matter, can do it for him.

*The Child Who Cannot Accept Responsibility for His Stuttering*

Some children seem to be unable to withstand the demands that are placed on them in therapy. Most Phase Four stutterers arrive at this level of difficulty in their teens—and adolescence is tough enough in itself. The child may be troubled with acne or scholastic or vocational worries; he may be anxious about relationships with the opposite sex, in addition to stuttering. When such additional sensitivities are present, the therapist will need to devote time to these troubles and will need to cement his relationship before he feels he can concentrate profitably on the stuttering. Some of these children may need a supportive type of therapy that will help them keep their heads above water until they can find it in themselves to work on their speech problem. It may be necessary to spend a greater than normal amount of time in explaining the basic logic of objectivity. It may be necessary to provide them with other types of help, such as vocational or educational counseling, before they feel strong enough to work responsibly on their speech.

With some stutterers it may be necessary to wait until the need to talk is imperative before they can assume responsibility for their own behavior. One youngster came to a willingness to work on his stuttering out of a feeling of guilt. His mother had broken her leg falling downstairs as she ran to answer the telephone. Instead of answering it himself, he had ducked into the next room when he heard it ring. The demands of earning a living may bounce a person out of the rut of relying on someone else to talk for him. One stutterer gained the necessary impetus in this manner:

My stuttering had bothered me for sometime, but never too seriously. Although I did not enjoy stuttering, and although I was sometimes laughed at because I stuttered, I did not feel greatly handicapped because of my speech difference. In school the teachers merely excused me from giving oral reports—a fact which I found somewhat advantageous. I dated easily and was elected "Most Popular Senior Boy." After high school, I felt fortunate to get a job as an operator for the railroad. My job was to call the chief dispatcher and report the arrival and departure times of all trains. I became so afraid of having to talk and my stuttering got so bad that they fired me. I sure don't like to use a shovel, but right now that's all I can find to do.

A second stutterer reported a less traumatic experience:

I didn't want to talk to anyone about my stuttering when I was younger. I guess I was real ashamed of it. I didn't even want to talk—period. My summer job in the grocery store just before my senior year in high school did the trick. I needed the money because I wanted to dress like the other guys. My folks couldn't afford it what with Dad being in the hospital for two months that spring. Man did I jump. I worked hard and was so tired sometimes that I could hardly drag myself home after work—especially on Saturday. But what got me was that nobody paid much attention to my stuttering. Some of the regular customers were real friendly and went out of their way to say "hello" to me. Somedays, especially when I had to load shelves, I was so bored I actually found myself starting conversation with some of the customers on my own. I had a real good boss. One day the boss asked me to answer the phone. Maybe he wasn't thinking and thought I was one of the other guys, but I felt real proud just the same when he asked me. I was scared and I stuttered too, but when I hung up I saw he was watching me. He just winked and I felt I'd pop my buttons.

Some children find it difficult to accept responsibility for their stuttering because their parents have assumed too much responsibility for their behavior. Some parents find it difficult to let their children grow up. They have hounded them for years about their speech and have told them what to do for it. The child enters therapy solely because his parents desire it. Such a child needs to receive assurance that help is available but therapy will not be forced down his throat. At the same time, however, the therapist should do what he can to let the child see that it is to *his* advantage to improve his speech. He may feel resentful toward his parents for continually reminding him of his problem, but he is the one who feels the most pain, the greatest embarrassment from the stuttering.

*Defining the Problem*

Many stutterers are unwilling to concentrate on their speech because to do so is to admit to something strange, something unknown, something dreaded. They rarely know much about others who stutter. To confess to stuttering is to admit that they are like those others who for some strange reason talk in strange ways. Who wants to confess to that much strangeness? Some don't mind thinking of what they do as "stammering" because stammering is somehow held to be a nicer, milder thing with a better prognosis than stuttering. Often "stuttering" is thought of as a condition "out of control" and irreversible. But the stutterer must be able to talk about his behavior and why it bothers him; he must be able to describe his worries and confess to their impact on him and how they affect his actions. Unless he can do this, he will find it extremely difficult to concentrate on the specific instances in which he stutters.

Because stuttering has always been such a dreaded thing to him, the stutterer may need to be shown how to talk about his problem. His therapist helps by the types of questions he asks. The questions direct the stutterer toward the kinds of things he needs to explore. But more than that, they show him a way to confront the problem. "What do you call what you are doing?" "How long has this been going on?" "Do you always talk as you are talking now?" "Does it change from time to time?" "What seems to make it change?"

The stutterer starts out falteringly, strongly feeling his incapability of confronting his problem, but, as he talks and tells, his therapist's reactions help dispel the threat of his confession. His therapist does not censor or pity. He acts as if he, for one, is on familiar ground. The nature of the questions begin to impress on the stutterer that the therapist has been over this ground before with others. Just as the stutterer has talked inwardly to himself, now he begins to talk outwardly about what it is like to stutter. As he talks about his stuttering, his reluctance to talk about it subsides. He has a good listener—one who does not try too hard to reassure and one who is not upset by what he hears. Although he is not told that his problem isn't so bad after all and is bearable, he begins to feel that way. The barrage of questions indicates the possibility of appropriate answers. The questions are probing. The therapist's most valuable tool at this point is "tell me more."

The client's early attempts to talk about his problem seem almost like a confession to him. He's been so ashamed of this problem for so long and has tried so hard to hide it for so long, that to describe it is like a confession to a "wrong." He has heard perhaps that "stutterers are neurotic" and so, when he openly talks about his stuttering, in a sense he is confessing to being a neurotic. It is important that the therapist begin work early to remove such emotional reactions. So long as the stutterer continues to think of his problem as akin to "sin" and requiring "confession," his attempts to work on his problem will continue to be focused on hiding the problem—on not committing the sin.

General semanticists have long stressed the fact that the words human beings use to describe their own "problem" behavior often turn out to be causing, contributing to, or maintaining the "problem." Johnson (3) and Williams (6) have applied this general semantics principle specifically to the problem of stuttering. According to this view, it makes a great deal of difference whether a person speaks of himself as a stutterer or as someone who stutters. As Williams states it:

> When a person begins thinking that a certain way of behaving is "part of him," or "just the way he is," it represents a relatively basic orientation that is reflected in the way he talks about himself. It implies that he is a certain kind of person. He believes that he may change certain ways of acting but that he cannot change the fundamental "him." In this context, the "him" seems to represent a special entity inside his body. This orientation is reflected in the attitude of a person who excuses himself from social activities by saying: "I can't meet people very well because I'm too shy." Yet, if one would ask him why he considers himself shy, he would likely answer that obviously he is shy because he can't meet people very well. By the use of such circular thinking he is talking and acting as if the attribute of "shyness" is inside of him and there is nothing he can do about it(6:391).

From this point of view then, it becomes important for the child to distinguish between "stuttering" and thinking of himself as a "stutterer." When therapists advocate that a child stop hiding his problem, they should not demand that he think of himself as a stutterer.* At the same time, however, it is important that a

---

* Speech therapists frequently find themselves in a quandary concerning

child be able to see his problem unemotionally and accept his differences for what they are. Since the advanced stutterer has tried so hard to hide his stuttering in the past and since his problem is charged with emotion, it may be quite difficult for him to accept his speech breakdowns. If a person feels sensitive about stumbling when walking and goes to great lengths to hide his stumbles by sitting as much as possible or walking behind others so they will not see him stumble, he needs to face up to his problem more directly before he can get over his fear of walking. He needs to accept his stumblings for what they are. But he does not necessarily gain anything; in fact, he will probably find his problem increased, if he begins to think of himself as a "stumbler."

A child needs a way to describe his stuttering objectively and hopefully. And there is a way to do so. According to Williams (6), a person who says he "stutters" talks about his "stuttering" as something that just happens because he is a "stutterer." When he gets a particular feeling in his stomach or in his chest this is a sign that "it" is about to happen. When he attempts to talk he tries to "hold the stuttering back" or to "get the words out without the stuttering coming out too." He views his stuttering as an entity, an animistic "thing" that lies inside him. The person doing the stuttering acts as if there is a little man inside him who grabs certain words, or he acts as if certain words are possessed of physical properties such that they get "stuck" in his throat. He equates what he does when he stutters with "it." "It," according to Williams, is a referent used by the stutterer to describe both cause and effect. This "it" being that undefinable "thing" that the stutterer has placed inside himself through the machinations of a special type of thinking. Thus, the stutterer thinks of his behavior as something *happening* to him rather than as something he *does*. Viewed from the standpoint of therapy, if something is "happening" to a person he cannot be expected to accept responsibility for his behavior because "it" is out of his power to control. Williams provides a valuable means of working through this dilemma. The person doing the stuttering is conscientiously urged

---

how they should refer to a person who stutters. Since they do not wish the client to adopt a self-image of "being a stutterer," they feel guilty when they use the term "stutterer." Suffice it to say, the label "stutterer" means different things to different people. To the therapist, this can be a convenient way to classify persons with similar problems. It does not need to imply anything more than that.

to monitor his verbal content and to frame statements about his behavior so that when he describes his behavior he accurately describes what he *does* and refrains from words that refer to something *happening* to him. He now is led to take responsibility for his lips and his tongue. Instead of "my lips wouldn't open" he is encouraged to report that he held his lips pressed tightly together. Instead of "my tongue was stuck" he describes his actions in terms of "I jammed my tongue hard against my upper teeth" or "I didn't move my tongue."

## Learning about Stuttering

The stutterer must remove "stuttering" from the land of the unknown where it seems to happen for its own mysterious reasons and repatriate it in the land of the identifiable where he is aware that he does something to make it happen. Once he realizes this, he learns a new way of thinking about his actions. His therapist shows him how it is possible for him to describe what he does when he "stutters" or what he does to keep from "stuttering." He is helped to describe his behavior more meaningfully. He is encouraged to refrain from using the word *stuttering* thoughtlessly. He is urged to describe what he does when he behaves in his "stuttering" way. Here is one example.

T: What did you do that time?
C: I stuttered real hard. That was like those I've been telling you about.
T: But what did you do?
C: My tongue sorta got stuck.
T: You got stuck? What did you do to get stuck?
C: I don't know what it was but the word wouldn't come out.
T: Were you pushing hard with your tongue?
C: Yes, my tongue was up against my top teeth. Just a little bit above there. It wouldn't move.
T: Did you try to move your tongue?
C: No, I couldn't. Well I didn't anyway.
T: Did you try to make a sound when you started to say the word?
C: No, my mouth was open but nothing came out.
T: Did you try to wiggle your jaw?
C: My lip went up and down some, yes.
T: What did you do just before you tried to say the word? Did you take a big breath and grunt?
C: Yes, that always happens.
T: Try it again. (*trial*) Now tell me what you did.

C: Well, I didn't grunt that time. But it kept going over and over.
T: What did?
C: The first part of the word.
T: You kept saying the first part of the word over and over?
C: I repeated it. Yes.
T: Where did you hold your tongue?
C: It locked right up tight again.
T: Where?
C: The same place.
T: You pushed hard and tight with your tongue. Did you try to move into the rest of the word?
C: After a while I could.
T: When did you think to move to the rest of the word?
C: Well, I didn't. My tongue just wouldn't budge. No. I jammed it real tight.

Note that this approach does not need to be confined to the most advanced stages of stuttering. This kind of description has value and meaning to children in the early stages of development. This approach, in modified form, was advocated in previous chapters.

## Removing the Stigma

Since so many stutterers have heard that they stutter because they were tickled as a baby, because they drank chocolate sodas, because they were "tongue-tied," or for some other equally false reason, it is important that misconceptions about the cause and nature of stuttering be cleared away. Some useful techniques for group therapy are: (a) Discussions may be conducted on the nature of "normal disfluencies" and their incidence in the speech of all persons. (b) Different stutterers may be asked to relate their ideas of stuttering causation and examine the rationale of these ideas in terms of present knowledge of speech production. These discussions need to be carefully guided and the therapist should actively teach, lead, and provide better information than the child formerly had access to. (c) The older child may look up easy-to-read explanations of stuttering etiology and the development of stuttering symptoms and use these readings as a basis for discussion in therapy sessions.

### Experiencing Stuttering

There is considerable consensus of opinion among speech pathologists that the growth of stuttering is based in large part on a stutterer's attempts to keep from stuttering. Phase Four stutterers, without prior treatment, may never have made a conscious attempt to stutter. Viewed in this context they have never really stuttered. Since all of their conscious efforts have been used to inhibit stuttering—to keep it from occurring, or to keep it from running away when it does occur—they have failed to learn what they do when they stutter because they were not stuttering but were trying to keep from stuttering.

As early as Phase Three and sometimes in Phase Two, the act of stuttering deliberately can contribute to a vastly different meaning of the behavior called stuttering. A psychological victory is scored when a child deliberately performs the tabooed act at the suggestion of his therapist. Instead of holding back he lets the stuttering stutter. He does it. Instead of feeling that he has failed because he was unable to hold the stuttering back he is now praised for letting it come out. Failure turns into success. By being permitted to stutter he learns that the act of stuttering, though punishing, is not the crux of his problem. He learns that what he does trying not to stutter keeps his tensions high and makes the act of stuttering so revolting to him. By actually stuttering, by faking, and by trying to make his tensions great enough to trigger a tremor, he learns to move ahead instead of oscillating between his urge to speak and his equally strong urge to remain silent. He finds that what he thought was dangerous and harmful is not so at all. He learns how to keep his wits about him when he is in what he considers dangerous territory. With his wits about him he can begin to look at what he is doing. He begins to feel power, a new kind of strength that he had denied himself before. He learns that to get over his stuttering he must stutter, but he now does it deliberately, consciously, purposefully.

He gains a new kind of freedom. Instead of his firmly held convictions that the only good stuttering was stuttering that didn't occur, that his audiences were justified in their intolerence of his stuttering, that he was wrong if he stuttered, he now actively engages in the thing he formerly actively avoided. Instead of being possessed by a dreaded affliction he now finds renewed pride in coping with his fears. Kent suggests that the therapist provide the following counsel:

> *Talk.* Do as much talking as you possibly can. Go out of your way to talk. If you find yourself backing away from something you are

afraid you *might* do, find out what you *do* do. When you make a "mistake," keep talking. This is what normal speakers do and this is one of the things you must practice doing in trying to do more of the things that normal speakers do when they talk. Talk to as many different people in as many different situations as possible. You have spent years learning to talk the way you do; you have talked in every conceivable situation. Do not be misled by accidental contingencies which might lead you to believe that you have discovered "a technique to make the stutter go away." There are no such techniques. Rather, concentrate on the discovery that stuttering is contingent only upon what you do. Although mistakes will be made when attempting to master some new behavior, these mistakes will, with continued constructive practice in a variety of situations, decrease in number and in degree to be replaced by a new desired behavior. You must strive for and look for improvement rather than a "cure."

*Be Afraid.* In the past you may have come to believe that "fear" in a situation inevitably results in your stuttering. This is a belief which should be tested. Although being afraid that you will stutter makes you uneasy, this fear alone cannot keep you from talking. Observe how many times you keep talking in spite of this fear of stuttering if you continue to do the things which are necessary in order to maintain the forward flow of speech, i.e., continue to move forward from one sound to the next. With practice you may find that you will improve in your ability to move forward from sound to sound and from word to word in spite of the fear that you will stutter. As you improve, you may find that more and more of the time you will be less and less afraid you will stutter.

*Be Embarrassed.* If people react to your speech in ways that embarrass you, be embarrassed, but keep talking. You have a problem just as almost everyone has a problem; unlike most people, however, you are doing something about yours. Being embarrassed cannot keep you from talking.

*Make Mistakes.* If you keep talking, you are bound to err occasionally. Everyone does. When you do, make yourself aware of precisely what you are doing that is interfering with the process of talking. Then, change what you are doing *while you are doing it* and keep talking (4:143-44).

## Other Concrete Actions

Often stutterers come into therapy bringing a history of self-denial, broken resolves, and unanswered prayers. Most often they have tried to help themselves by trying not to stutter, manfully, through brute effort and stern resolve. Some try wishful thinking. Very few have worked systematically with a plan. Most have tried will power, and autosuggestion. They have tried to follow the advice of well-wishers who have said, "All you have to do is . . ." Usually their advisor is well-intentioned but ill-informed. They are told that they should not worry about what others think (and so they learn an exaggerated concern for their listeners and learn to worry more about the effect of their stuttering on others.) Or they are encouraged to concentrate on the times when they are at ease and relaxed and they are urged to try to remain calm in certain difficult situations—"Because really no one will bite you!" (Try to be determined to be relaxed! Determination and relaxation simply do not go together.) Many report that they get up in the morning determined not to stutter and, subsequently defeated, they go to bed that night praying for the fortitude and necessary strength to hide their panic, humiliation, and disillusionment the next day.

Therapy provides a way of attacking problems which assures a better approach to a solution than sheer will power. This new approach sets relief from stuttering as a final goal. But instead of concentrating on that last final goal it urges establishment of attainable subgoals. These subgoals enable the child to be realistic about what he needs to do to re-establish fluency, beginning considerably away from fluency and working toward it one step at a time.

At first the stutterer may need to acknowledge the fact that, although he habitually tries not to stutter, when he does stutter he usually tries to ignore it. In order to face his stuttering he must know when he stutters and he must be able to recognize when he does it. He should be able to collect instances of stuttering. Between sessions he can write down words he has stuttered until he collects 50 or 450 stuttered words depending on the quota set either by himself or his therapist. Now he is doing something concrete. He has something to report, something specific to concentrate on. He has a daily set of things to accomplish. He has a way of achieving while "failing." Up until this time he has regretted every moment of stuttering, feeling that every time he stutters he has failed to keep his promise to himself. When he counts the times he stutters for a purpose, for example, to determine whether he stutters more in some situations than others, he begins to know something objective about his stuttering. He can begin to change the vocabulary he used to describe his stuttering episodes. Instead of saying, "I stuttered an awful lot in French class," he can now say, "I stuttered on seven different words in French class. I was able to look up at my instructor, before I looked down at my book to read. The first word I stuttered on I said over and stuttered on it again the second time, but I said it again anyway even though I knew I would stutter."

Energies needed to combat stuttering should not be misspent trying to 'conceal stuttering. Most therapies allow an opportunity for the stutterer to tell about his stuttering first to his therapist, then to others, and finally to audiences of various sizes. They are encouraged to tell their friends what they do in therapy. They are required to learn about stuttering so they can teach others about it. But they are also encouraged to clear the air for themselves and the people to whom they speak. Thus, at various times they are encouraged to say things such as, "Let me try that word again. I sure butchered it." Or "That one sure got away from me." They are encouraged to look at the people to whom they are talking and to indicate that although they are having trouble talking they are trying to learn to do something about it.

### Changing the Response

Once the stutterer has learned to experience stuttering instead of running away from it, he is ready to begin changing his reaction to the anticipation and act of stuttering. There are several key parts to changing the stutterer's response: (a) he can learn to inhibit certain signs of excess tension associated with the attempt to overcome stuttering; (b) he can change those behaviors which lead to undesirable audience responses; and (c) he may develop a tolerance for his speech failures so that they do not become cues for renewed tension. The first point, i.e., inhibiting the signs of excess tension, was covered in detail in Chapter Five. The stutterer needs to learn a new set of behaviors in place of his former tense, disorganized attempts to produce speech. Viewed in terms of a drive-reduction theory of learning and with the well-known stimulus-response bond in mind, stuttering at the Phase Four level may be thought of as a set of behaviors learned in response to the stimulus of speech anxiety. Much of the anxiety should already be reduced by this stage of therapy due to his newfound ability to talk about his stuttering. According to drive-reduction theory, the response is learned in association with the drive. When the drive (in this case, the anxiety) is completely absent, the response of becoming overly tense, repeating words, and otherwise displaying behaviors which we call stuttering will probably not be evoked. When the stutterer feels anxious about speaking, the learned responses (stuttering) will be evoked unless they have been unlearned and new substitute responses learned in association with the drive. Therapy needs to be directed not only at decreasing the stimulus of speech anxiety which produces the stuttering but toward helping the stutterer learn new responses at those times when he does feel anxious, especially since one can never be completely rid of anxiety. The best way we know to help a child modify his response is by the use of cancellations, pull-outs, and preparatory sets. Since these were explained in Chapter Five, further elaboration will not be made here except to point out that the child needs to be willing to experiment with these various steps and the accompanying techniques in order for the changes in response to occur. Although the principles of modifying the response are the same, the Phase Four stutterer may exhibit considerably more difficulty than the Phase Three stutterer in attempting the modifications since his self-concept of being "a stutterer" is more strongly fixed and since his stuttering behaviors have been learned over a longer period of time and are accompanied by a greater degree of anxiety.

## Changing the Listener's Response

One of the factors which perpetuates the stutterer's anxiety and therefore his stuttering is his anticipation of undesirable reactions from those who hear him stutter. Doubtlessly, the stutterer has received some unfavorable audience reactions during the history of his stuttering. Because of those he has received, he expects to receive more. He is constantly on guard, suspecting unfavorable reactions, and he frequently misinterprets the reactions of others to his stuttering. He may sense pity when none is there. He may inaccurately project rejection when the true reaction of the listener is closer to bewilderment. Often he accurately senses that his listeners are concerned about the way he talks, but he misjudges the direction of their concern or feels unable to do anything about unfavorable reactions which he does receive. Therapy must help the stutterer to learn about the predicament of the listener. The stutterer should learn that the reaction he observes in others may be based on healthy curiosity instead of studied condescension and that any embarrassment observed may be due to the listener's lack of knowledge concerning how the speaker prefers to be treated. The "perceived condescension" may be a truly earnest effort to refrain from offending. The stutterer's listeners often do not know what to do when confronted with stuttering. They know they do not want to patronize or to pry. They don't want to offend by unsolicited sympathy. Nor does the stutterer know what to do. Before therapy, he rarely acknowledged his stuttering even when he stuttered most. He struggled vainly through his faltering facsimile of conversation while his listener, polite but bewildered, pretended calm, a posture devoid of helpful response on either side. Thus, both the stutterer and his auditor, engaged in a comedy of manners, remained deadlocked in a cacophonous calamity. The stutterer needs to learn that he is the key figure in these dramatic encounters because he is in a better position to put his listener at ease than his listener is to put him at ease.

The stutterer needs to understand the listener's dilemma. He can learn to help his listener by indicating his own recognition of a particularly tough word with such phrases as, "Wow, I really hung up on that one. Let me try it again." The stutterer can show his own awareness of the amusing facet of some of his blocks by displaying them, wherever appropriate, so that he too can laugh at stuttering. The stutterer can change the response of the listener by maintaining normal eye contact when talking and by not becoming so flustered that he makes his listener feel pity. Analogies are helpful here. If the stutterer can learn the difference between a display of severe embarrassment as compared to humorous open acceptance of an embarrassing slip of the tongue, then he is in a better position to know how to react when his stuttering has humorous aspects. One of our collegiate stutterers told us this story:

> I went into the telephone office one morning bright and early to pay a past-due bill. I was embarrassed about being tardy in my account and thought I had better apologize for it. I was all set to do this, but just as I started to say something, the young clerk behind the desk asked, "How are you?" For some reason—maybe it was because it was early in the morning or maybe it was because I hadn't expected her question, it threw me off and I began to stutter. "I-I-I-I'm a month late," then quickly remembered her question and added "How are you?" The way my questions came out made us both slightly flustered, but she rose to the occasion quickly and

responded with a laugh, "I'm fine, thank you, but don't worry, you'll be the first to know if anything changes."

We agree with others who feel it helps the stutterer to be able to tell jokes about his stuttering. As he becomes better able to laugh at himself, he prevents adverse audience reactions by not becoming completely embarrassed when his stuttering does have a comical side. Even though it is not desirable for the stutterer to feel that his speech problem is something to be laughed at, he needs to know that everyone at times pulls embarrassing slips. The ability to recognize when they should be openly admitted and when it is advantageous to continue without apparent recognition can add considerably to the speaker's poise.

### Accepting Less than Perfection

Another side to objectivity which must not be overlooked concerns the ability of a stutterer to tolerate his failures in therapy. Many stutterers, once they have gained some degree of relief from stuttering, seem to forget that avoidances and uncontrolled blocks were formerly their most consistent stuttering symptoms. When they find themselves reverting to the old habitual patterns, they feel as if their progress has been lost. A severe block early in the morning may make them so upset that the frequency and severity of their stuttering is increased for the rest of the day. This one act of stuttering sets off increased tension, increased stuttering, and increased avoidance behavior.

Stutterers need to learn that such relapses have to be accepted as normal. There will always be difficult days. There will be many instances when the severity of their stuttering is increased. The stutterer needs to accept the fact that no one can be perfect. He also needs to know that he can pick himself up after falling down. A severe stuttering block on one word does not have to be the forerunner of increased stuttering. The use of an avoidance mechanism does not necessarily mean that all of the old fear has returned.

Perhaps one reason stutterers fear relapse is that they are still afraid that stuttering might not be controllable. If such is the case, the therapist might find it useful to arrange for the stutterer to experience a great deal of success in handling his most feared words. Another approach is to ask the stutterer to try to get himself into uncontrollable blocks and prolong them as long as possible. The act of prolonging a block almost invariably brings it under voluntary control, thus demonstrating to him that his fears are ungrounded.

The basic lesson to be taught is that the child can learn a new set of responses to the same stimuli which formerly set off the secondary stuttering behaviors. The stimuli leading to increased anxiety can be partially decreased, but the responses to the stimuli can be altered by modifying the excess tension in the speech musculature, by acting in such a way as to create better audience reactions, and by learning that the abnormality caused by increased tension on one word or in one situation does not have to transfer to all other words and situations.

## Providing for Reinforcement

New responses not only must occur, they must also be reinforced. For our purposes here, those rewards provided by the therapist, such as praise, will be termed "indirect rewards." The stutterer needs to gain some kind of reward for the performance of his new responses to speech anxiety. If he is not rewarded in some way, the new responses will not become automatic, as exemplified by the following incident related by a student clinician.

> I don't know what to do about Ed. After several sessions where we discussed how avoidance increases fear and fear increases stuttering, he seemed to be willing to enter speaking situations which he used to avoid. But after a couple of days of appearing to get the idea, he now refuses to do any assignments. Do you know what he said to me today? He said, "I always have gotten by without having to talk to people, why should I start doing it now?"

As the therapist discussed this with her supervisor, it became apparent that the stutterer was not yet receiving any direct rewards for stuttering openly and the therapist was failing to provide the proper kind of indirect rewards. The more the child entered his feared situations, the more the therapist pointed out to him how afraid he was. As a result, the old response of not talking to people seemed far better to Ed than did the new response—especially when his only reinforcement was in being told how afraid he was.

When a stutterer is first trying out the new responses, it is particularly important that the therapist provide indirect rewards for these attempts. The rewards may be in the form of praise and encouragement. The rewards may consist of verbal recognition that the stutterer has done something which took a great deal of courage. The rewards may come simply from doing something which the child feels is pleasing his therapist. One reason the child needs more indirect reinforcement during his early attempts to carry out feared speech tasks is that his tension is probably high and his stuttering is likely to be more severe. As he enters more difficult situations and these experiences become less traumatic, the child is able to provide his own rewards. When he finds that audience reactions are more favorable during those instances where he goes directly into his feared words instead of using postponement devices, he is directly rewarded and thus encouraged to do more of the same. When he successfully employs loose contact on a feared word, his behavior is reinforced. The direct reinforcement he receives from reduced anxiety and increased confidence in speaking is now much more beneficial than the indirect rewards provided by the therapist. The therapist's praise may help to encourage the child to attempt something he has been afraid to try, but these attempts will not become learned responses unless direct rewards are received.

## The Assignment Method

A valuable tool to help concretize therapy and to provide for both direct and indirect reinforcement is available through the use of assignments. Ideally these are devised by the child himself or through a cooperative effort with his therapist. In the beginning stages of therapy the therapist usually provides the assignments, using guide-lines such as these.

*Assignments should be meaningful.* They should help the child to learn something about himself and about his stuttering. They should not be busywork assignments but should be related to predetermined goals.

*Assignments should be specific.* They should be stated so that the child knows what he is to do, and how much he has or has not accomplished.

*Assignments should be reportable.* A good assignment will enable the child to report in specific terms what he has done.

*Assignments should be verifiable.* The therapist should be able to check on whether and how well the assignment was fulfilled. *Assignments should be reasonable.* The assignment must be assured of a reasonable chance for success and must be something that could be reasonably required of the child.

Bloodstein has this to say about assignments:

> Whatever methods are used to eliminate avoidances and teach the stutterer that stuttering is not so fearful, the projects or assignments which he undertakes should be specific, clearly defined, and capable of evaluation in terms of success or failure, a rule which applied to other phases of stuttering therapy as well. In addition, it is of the utmost importance to keep in mind two related principles having broad application to the planning and evaluation of the stutterer's work in outside situations. The first is never to assume that simply because we have told the stutterer clearly and repeatedly what we believe he must do and why, he has an adequate understanding of what we mean. The second is to assume that once we have listened to the stutterer's account of the experiences he has had, the observations he has made, and the things he has accomplished or failed to accomplish, we have a rough idea of what he was talking about. Anyone who ignores these precepts will almost certainly receive some jarring surprises before he learns to demonstrate to the stutterer as far as possible what he means and to observe the stutterer as far as possible as he does it (1:50-51).

The assignment method is advantageous in that the essential responsibility is on the stutterer himself—not the therapist. It takes therapy out of the realm of "just talking" and reinforces insight with appropriate action. Therapy procedures inevitably become more meaningful and easier to accomplish if they are stated in meaningful terms so that they can be attempted for a reason and within reasonable limits. Failures can be pinpointed. Success can be measured. When alterations in plans need to be made, the child's performance can be used as a basis for the alterations. Especially important is the fact that the child himself will know how well he is doing. The child wants to grow and change. He will do what he is ready to do. The therapist by using specific assignments can help fractionate the child's behavior appropriately so that the child can find out what he is ready to accomplish. By careful design the child can discover success without stumbling on it by chance through trial-and-error attempts to change himself.

It is wise to allow the child an opportunity to choose his own time for change. He may help in planning and setting up specific assignments. The first several assignments will of necessity need to be set up in advance to show how they should be done. After he performs them he will know what they can help him accomplish. Sometimes a child is ready to change but reluctant to brave an attempt at a new type of behavior. He may be given several assignments, some easier than others but aimed at the same goal. This will force a decision toward the needed change, but the decision will be his.

### Self-Understanding

As stated earlier in this chapter, no one can really view any aspect of himself in a completely detached or unemotional manner. Neither can anyone completely understand himself. Indeed, the rarest of our species and sometimes the most unfortunate are those who know themselves too well. Although theoretically self-understanding leads to adjustment, the process of understanding self as a means to adjustment is not always productive. Adjustment is an abstract word intended to describe a desirable state of being. Preoccupation with the achievement of adjustment often prevents its occurrence, especially when the ledger of self-understanding ends up with more debits than credits, more liabilities than assets, more failures than successes.

What has been written so far concerning the objective attitude and the therapy plan for the Phase Four stutterer implies that he should know himself and his stuttering. Specifically, he should understand that, regardless of the original instigator, stuttering is perpetuated by what he has done and is doing. It may be that what he has done has come about by accident out of ignorance or even stupidity. Well-meaning friends and relatives may also have added to his storehouse of poor attitudes, wrong responses, and misconceptions. But although what he has done may have helped him into a pattern of behavior that is difficult to change, he should realize that this well-established pattern can be altered or broken and a new, more rewarding behavior can emerge. He needs to know about himself because he needs to know how his strengths and weaknesses have contributed to his stuttering. He needs to take stock. He may profit from writing his autobiography. In it he can describe his family, his friends, his schooling, his physical appearance. He should list his assets and liabilities, what he has accomplished and what he needs to accomplish.*

The therapist can help the stutterer in his self-understanding by giving assignments, by being a good listener, and by the direction he provides during therapy discussions. Assignments can be planned which focus the stutterer's attention on aspects of his behavior which the therapist feels are important for him to notice. One stutterer, a college co-ed, was helped to see that her stuttering was simply one small facet of a general tendency to become disorganized and flustered under stress situations. Over a period of months, the student presented a running series of emotional upsets. The causes of the traumatic incidents varied—breaking up with a boy friend, not being understood by her parents, difficulty in course work, and damaging a fender on the boy friend's car—but the essential pattern stayed the same. She would feel threatened, would become anxious, would "panic" and be unable to handle the problem without help. Her stuttering history was quite similar. She would readily learn how to control a particular stuttering symptom, but when she encountered a severe stuttering block, she would panic and feel unable to solve the problem by herself. In all of these instances, the threat of a speech block or of a personal problem led to random, disorganized attempts to handle the situation. As the individual therapy sessions continued, the therapist gradually helped her to see the similarity between feeling blocked in speech and feeling blocked in personal difficulties. As she developed a better understanding of her over-all pattern of behavior and of her need to be dependent on others, she was able to prevent the development of extreme anxiety and the consequent random behavior. This increase in self-understanding led to more

---

* *Self-Inventory* and *Know Yourself* are workbooks which offer systematic means for making these necessary self-assessments. These workbooks are suited to Junior High School and High School students. The stated purpose of *Self-Inventory* is to seek to bring out into the open that which some children try to hide. *Know Yourself* is a personal workbook for those who stutter. These spiral-bound books provide specific ratings of attitudes toward stuttering, adjustment quizzes, means for the child to describe the way he stutters, and many other concrete opportunities for a child to know himself and his stuttering.

Bryng Bryngelson, Myfanwy E. Chapman, and Orvetta K. Hansen, *Know Yourself: A Workbook for Those Who Stutter,* Third Ed. (Minneapolis: Burgess Publishing Company, 1958).

Myfanwy E. Chapman, *Self-Inventory: Group Therapy for Those Who Stutter,* Third Ed. (Minneapolis: Burgess Publishing Co., 1959).

suitable adjustments of personal problems as well as to better control of speech behaviors.

## The Products of Therapy

The final goal of therapy might be described as spontaneity in speech. Fluency in speaking is an outward manifestation of spontaneity. Fluency has been described before in several ways but is usually equated with the relatively imperfect fluency of most normal speakers. Fluency is effortless speech unmarred by tensions, tremors, or repetitions. The fluency sought by the therapist for the child with whom he is working is not perfect fluency, but reasonable fluency—fluency that is tolerant of occasional stumbles and blunders—fluency that is not inhibited by a lack of self-confidence. Therapy procedures should provide for the development of greater fluency and for the reinforcement of fluency in a variety of circumstances. The next chapter takes up the terminal phases of therapy and this important topic will be enlarged upon there.

Equally important with the development of fluency is the emergence of a new self-concept. The Phase Four stutterer brings into therapy a set of values and judgments which help to set off and maintain his stutterings. Because he is unaware of the mental mechanisms he employs, his behavior is perpetuated. Therapy procedures concentrate on eliminating fears and their by-products, and in the process attitudes and self-concepts change. The child is urged to see not only his shortcomings but his positive attributes and achievements, and, as he opens his eyes to the positive side of himself, he grows in dignity and confidence. He no longer feels that what he does is unworthy of himself and undeserving of the respect of others.

Along with these attitude changes, the child learns a philosophy that change is possible. He learns to do first things first and to experiment with his behavior. This experimentation helps him to become less rigid, less inclined to behave always in the same way. As he is freed from his morbid concern with whether he can say what he wants to say, he is less and less inclined to let rust form on his talking tools. He seeks out situations in which he can talk, at first with the guidance of his clinician, but eventually on his own.

As he enjoys the ready freedom of talk, he creates opportunities to talk. The barbershop is no longer a fearful place; he finds new interest in the person sitting next to him in class; he says "hello" cheerfully to people he meets on the street; he uses the telephone; he talks—spontaneously—as he should. He learns the pleasure of society, comradeship, small talk, the relaxation of quiet conversation at the corner drug store. This is his motivation and goal and as he rejoins society on an equal footing, the therapist is rewarded.

## References

1. BLOODSTEIN, O. "Stuttering as an Anticipatory Struggle Reaction," In J. Eisenson (ed.) *Stuttering: A Symposium* (New York: Harper & Row, Publishers, 1958).
2. DOLLARD, J. and N. E. MILLER. *Personality and Psychotherapy* (New York: McGraw-Hill Book Company, Inc., 1950).
3. JOHNSON, W. *People in Quandaries* (New York: Harper & Row, Publishers, 1946).
4. KENT, L. R. "A Retraining Program for the Adult Who Stutters," *Journal of Speech and Hearing Disorders*, XXVI (1961), 141-44.
5. VAN RIPER, C. *Speech Correction: Principles and Methods*, Fourth Ed. (Englewood Cliffs, N.J.: Prentice-Hall, Inc., 1963).
6. WILLIAMS, D. E. "A Point of View About Stuttering," *Journal of Speech and Hearing Disorders*, XXII (1957), 390-97.

# Chapter Seven

## The Termination of Therapy

*This chapter is concerned with the final outcome of therapy and the child's consequent dismissal from therapy. Termination policies necessarily differ from one developmental phase to another. Although fluency is important, fluency, per se, is not the only criterion upon which a decision to terminate therapy is based.*

The termination of therapy is in reality a transfer of responsibility. Responsibility once partially invested in the therapist is fully reassumed by the child, the parent, and perhaps the child's teacher. This shift may take place gradually or suddenly, permanently or temporarily, systematically or in a disorganized manner. Therapy may terminate successfully and it may end in disappointment. The more involved the therapy, the more it is important to have an organized ending to the therapeutic relationship.

Termination does not necessarily imply a cure. There may be many different reasons for deciding to bring therapy to a close. Therapy may be terminated either by the therapist or by the client. Hopefully, both will be involved in the decision. From the standpoint of the therapist, many of the reasons for ending regular sessions may be found in this statement by one group of speech pathologists:

Treatment may be discontinued:
1. When the stutterer feels sufficiently self-confident in his ability to speak and the clinician agrees that this feeling is justified.
2. When, during the initial interview or in the course of therapy, it becomes obvious that the person is severely disturbed emotionally. In this case, referral for psychiatric consultation should be arranged.
3. When no satisfactory therapeutic relationship can be achieved or when the results of therapy continue over a substantial period to be unsatisfactory. In this case, referral to another speech clinician may be indicated.
4. When a level of improvement has been reached beyond which further progress appears unlikely.
5. When the stutterer has developed a sufficient degree of tolerance for such stuttering as he may continue to do after maximum improvement has been reached.
6. When the stutterer feels certain, and the clinician agrees, that he will be able to continue to improve without further supervision or assistance (3:31).

At times, therapy may be discontinued by extenuating circumstances having little to do with the child's speech progress. For example, the child may move from one school district to another and thus be no longer available for therapy. Sometimes scheduling conflicts with other activities necessitate an end to therapy. In some instances, the child decides for himself when the worst is past and his stuttering is no longer a problem. How soon he arrives at this decision—aside from progress in therapy—will depend on his attitudes, his standards of fluency, and his ability to be tolerant of himself and his disfluencies. The signal indicating that the time has arrived for the beginning of the end of therapy may come when the child feels that his blocks are no longer inevitable.

The therapist, however, should have a say in the final decision, if only to concur. It is not always easy to know when therapy should be discontinued because the line dividing normal speech and stuttered speech is neither clean-cut nor easy to trace. Siegenthaler, Davis, and Christensen (5) demonstrated that speech status and the therapist's recommendations for the continuance of speech therapy are not related to each other. Attitudes, both optimistic and realistic, play a part. Siegenthaler and Flamm (4) have shown that the therapist and stutterer are not likely to agree on how much progress has been made in therapy. Often the person receiving the therapy decides that sessions are no longer necessary before his therapist reaches the same conclusion.

### Preterminal Activities

Ideally, therapy will be completed in a careful, systematic manner. Due to the strength of the relationship that builds up during long-term stuttering therapy sessions, some weaning—some modification of activities—is usually necessary. Children become dependent on their therapist despite steps taken by the latter to prevent such attachment. Even when close emotional ties are not present, the child or parent is likely to transfer a good bit of the responsibility to the therapist. Sudden, unplanned termination of therapy may result in a loss of confidence and subsequent relapse. The answer lies in carrying out preterminal activities aimed at building safeguards to prevent possible pitfalls.

### Storehouse of Successful Speech Experiences

When termination is being considered, the therapist should arrange for the child to have many opportunities to enter speech situations where his speech performance will be successful and where he will be provided with positive rewards. This is not to say that the child should always be expected to give public performances before strangers to demonstrate his new-found skill. Frequently such appearances merely increase tension. The Phase One stutterer may experience his rewards simply by talking easily in situations where he formerly exhibited excessive disfluencies. The Phase Four stutterer may find renewed interest in speech from his ability to carry on conversations with strangers. The point to be remembered is that the therapist has the responsibility for seeing that success is experienced in many different situations. Regardless of whether such activities are planned or merely come about in the normal course of events, the therapist should check the child's speech and ensure that the proper kinds of rewards are being received.

### *Reviewing What Has Been "Learned"*

One of the most useful techniques for helping an individual reassume authority for his or his child's speech behavior is to summarize the problem as it was at the beginning of therapy and as it has changed. Those aspects of behavior and attitudes which should be continued or guarded against may be emphasized. If a parent has been inclined to expect perfection in his child's behavior, he needs to be reminded of the possibility of a return to this kind of undesired expectation. If an older stutterer has learned to stop hiding his stuttering, he should be reminded of the reasons for continuing to do so.

The child or the parent can learn much from verbalizing the major factors leading to an increase of speech tension and how they went about solving the problem. The changes that take place during therapy are often so gradual that the individual forgets he has made them. Reinforcement through reverbalization helps to fixate the progress that has been made.

#### Criteria for Successful Termination of Therapy

The end of therapy should not be dependent solely upon school schedules or the convenience of the parents. Therapy should be terminated when it appears that progress can be continued without the therapist's help. The reduction of the frequency of stutterings is not always a meaningful signal for the end of therapy. When stuttering symptoms abate or disappear it must be determined whether the remission is temporary or permanent. When stuttering symptoms suddenly and dramatically disappear, especially when therapy has been underway for only a short time, the symptoms can be expected to return. Assurance of a permanent change in speech patterns must be based on a genuine reduction of anxiety and apprehension concerning the act of stuttering. When a residue of stuttering remains in a person's speech the therapist must estimate the person's insight, ingenuity, and general response to therapy procedures in order to conclude with confidence that the person can manage to improve without too much additional professional guidance. The difficulty at arriving at a sure decision is stressed by Ainsworth:

> It has been the policy of the writer to retain the records of a stutterer in the inactive files for several years after specific treatment has stopped. At present, there are no reliable means of determining when a stutterer is "cured." Thus, in the sense that we use it with articulatory cases, he cannot be legitimately dismissed as satisfactory even though his speech is generally adequate. This does not mean that a stutterer needs to be a chronic attender of the speech class. On the contrary, he should be encouraged to go out on his own as soon as the clinician can be reasonably certain that such a procedure will not result in deterioration. . . .
>
> For the purpose of record keeping, a stutterer may be listed as satisfactory if he has had reasonably fluent speech for one year, but there should always be the qualification that the stuttering may return (1:105-6).

## Criteria for Dismissing the Incipient Stutterer

The most important indication of the successful effects of therapy with the beginning stutterer is the understanding displayed by the child's parents and teachers. When the important adults in the child's environment show by their reactions and comments that they realize the part played by fear, tension, and perfectionism in the problem of stuttering, termination may be considered. When this understanding is backed up by objective proof that communicative pressures are recognized and modified, that an ameliorative emotional climate has been established, and that overt reactions to the child's disfluencies no longer increase the child's awareness of his speech difficulty, a successful conclusion to therapy may be predicted more confidently.

The therapist should feel confident that the beginning stutterer's parents understand completely the preventive aspects of therapy. They should know that at this stage successful therapy means the prevention of more severe forms of stuttering and of more involved emotional attitudes toward speech, that fear and embarrassment in speaking are not usually present in the beginning stutterer and can be prevented from developing.

Although fluency in speaking is not the only determiner of successful speech therapy, it is definitely the focus of the problem and needs to be evaluated. The therapist will want to verify the absence of frequent stutterings, especially those accompanied by excessive tension. This evaluation is often difficult due to the episodic nature of stuttering at this stage. Over a period of time, however, it should become evident that the child's disfluencies are becoming less and less frequent and less severe.

### The Transitional Stutterer

Since the transitional stutterer is beginning to think of himself as a person who has difficulty in talking, a change in this aspect of his self-image should be achieved before therapy is discontinued. Definite evidence of an improvement in the child's concept of his own ability to talk should be sought. If he is old enough to have acquired a strong image of himself as a "stutterer," this opinion should be modified to the point where the child realizes that stuttering is something he "used to do" or "sometimes does" but which is neither grossly abnormal nor permanent.

In addition to the attitudinal changes, the Phase Two stutterer should display a real difference in the common form of his disfluencies. The tense, hard contacts which are characteristic of the transitional stutterer should be reduced in number and those that still remain replaced by easier, more relaxed repetitions and prolongations. Parents and teachers should understand that effortless disfluencies are signs of progress. They should also recognize the importance of their own roles in the development and attainment of secure spontaneous speech for their child.

### The Confirmed Stutterer

The criteria for the more advanced stages of stuttering will include all of the factors considered important for the earlier stages. In addition, the decision to end therapy in the case of the Phase Three stutterer should be based on the elimination of associated mannerisms. Particular attention should be paid to the removal of release and starter devices. The stutterer should not only have eliminated these crutches but should understand the dangers involved in their use.

Specific attention should be paid to the amount of fear that is attached to specific difficult words or situations. If the child still views many speech experiences as too difficult for him and still expects to stutter in them, he should remain in therapy.

Since the confirmed stutterer is generally highly aware of being a stutterer, he should not be dismissed until it is evident that this self-concept has been eliminated or greatly modified. Since there has been considerable controversy concerning whether a person who was once a "stutterer" but who has successfully completed therapy should continue to think of himself as a "stutterer," this point bears further discussion. At the termination of therapy for a very young child, not much question about his status need remain. For all intents and purposes he is a normal speaker. His reputation has been successfully changed from one who stuttered to one who at one time tended to stutter. The same applies to the Phase Two stutterer, but because he has stuttered longer his reputation as a "stutterer" is better established and more difficult to shake. What about Phase Three and Phase Four stutterers? Are they still stutterers? Some of them will discontinue their therapy with a residue of stuttering marring their speaking pattern. Most of them will not have eradicated all of their memories of unpleasant stuttering experiences. They may have terminated therapy with a new set of attitudes to fortify them under adverse speaking situations, but relapses into occasional tremors and unconscious avoidances are seldom completely eliminated.

Some therapists advocate that when the stutterer thinks of himself as a "stutterer," it helps him to exercise caution about his status as a speaker. By reminding himself that the trap of avoidance behavior is omnipresent, he is less apt to find himself completely off guard. He is better able to defend himself against the encroachment of subtle rephrasing of words because of a tiny flash of his old remembered fear of words and situations. He may be able to resist the blandishments of those who assure him that he has completely licked his problem. He can take pride in being a "well-adjusted stutterer," such as this case illustrates:

I truly am what I am! I stutter, so what? I am not afraid to admit
it. I have it well under control. I can maintain the delicate balance
necessary to maintain a gratifying level of self-esteem. I do not have
to repress what appears to you to be stuttering-like behaviors—at
least I don't have to repress them out of the fear of the consequences, nor do I have to flaunt my stutterings at you out of
bravado. I display just enough of what I do when I stutter that
I will be accepted and given responsibility on the basis of my true
everyday speaking performance. When I stutter I do so because of
outside pressures and disturbances over which I cannot exert too
much control. I expect that to happen. Most important to me and
my self-confidence is that I can account for periodic increases in the
frequency of my stutterings without undue worry.

This attitude or insight may work well for one person but not
another. Another person may find it discouraging to view himself
as a stutterer. Old ghosts of penalties, imagined or real, may come
back to haunt him simply because he is not permitted actively to
forget. Echoes of past word and situation failures may cause him
to cringe or pull his punches on some words involuntarily. Some
of his reactions may be way out of proportion to his felt need to
defend himself and he may find it in himself to be disappointed,
chagrined, or embarrassed about his "failings." His off-guard moments keep him on the sharp edge of frustration. He may permit
himself tiny subterfuges, an ever increasing quota of his old dodges
and avoidance devices to maintain his façade of a well-adjusted
stutterer. He may need to keep his emotions pitched unusually
high to maintain an objective attitude as a cover-up to hide from
himself and others his deep-seated, even basic anxiety about
whether he can really talk.

Some stutterers should be encouraged to continue to refer to
themselves as stutterers and to their speech as stuttered. Some
should not. The fact of remission of symptoms is well known. This
is especially true of the Phase Four stutterer. These people have
stuttered enough to be thoroughly shaken by their experiences.
They have been severely traumatized by their stuttering and their
urgency to get over their stuttering. Their desire to obtain true
freedom from stuttering is real and completely dominates their
thinking. Many have been demoralized by their stuttering and
are so traumatized that they cannot adjust their self-concept to
one compatible with that of being a nonstutterer. These people

need to find a way that will assure them lasting freedom from the threat of stuttering.

Some want freedom from stuttering so badly that they will take any kind of fluency as a token of their freedom. They need to be cautioned that they are not yet out of the woods. Because they are willing to employ self-deception to assure themselves that a cure is obtainable and that they have found it, they may cling tenaciously to the first device or technique that unlocks fluency. Some resist further therapy after achieving fluency so as to be able to disassociate themselves from anything that is a reminder of stuttering. It is especially important that the therapist arrange for follow-up visits—that the door is left open for a return to regular sessions when stuttering returns—which invariably happens.

Most Phase Three stutterers however can be dissuaded from accepting a permanent label of "stutterer" without experiencing undue adjustment difficulties. To them, stuttering generally failed to become a serious personal problem and consequently did not so completely affect their lives. Often the child himself makes the decision concerning the permanence of the label. Unless the therapist feels strongly that avoidances and increased tension will result from dropping the label "stutterer" no attempt should be made to insist on its remaining.

Whether or not the person feels he should retain a label of stutterer, the therapist must prompt his client to accept the responsibility of "working on his speech" outside of the therapy sessions. Also, he must understand that he speaks more fluently only when he does more of the things a normal speaker does and fewer of the things he has learned to do which interfere with the forward flow of speech (2).

## The Advanced Stutterer

Complete freedom from stuttering is not a reasonable goal for the advanced stutterer. It is realistic, however, to seek a reduction of the abnormality and tension accompanying the stuttering. The Phase Four stutterer can learn to exercise control over the majority of his stutterings. He can and should learn to prevent major portions of his secondary behaviors. He should also be expected to know what to do when he experiences considerable stuttering.

He should no longer have a feeling of complete hopelessness when he encounters a difficult word.

Perhaps the most important goal for the advanced stutterer is a change in his attitude of being handicapped. So long as the stutterer retains feelings of being different, he will experience excess tension in his contacts with others. This excess tension will counteract any control he attempts to exert and will maintain both the frequency and severity of his blocks. To feel handicapped is to be handicapped. One can accept a label of "stutterer" without feeling handicapped.

The advanced stutterer cannot be considered successfully rehabilitated unless he has reduced his avoidance devices to a minimum and has developed a strong conscience against employing techniques to hide his stuttering. Even though he may tolerate occasional lapses in the use of avoidances, his basic attitude should demonstrate his understanding of the dangers involved in their use and a willingness to face what is temporarily difficult in order to achieve a more desirable long-term goal.

The Phase Four stutterer should have demonstrated the ability to eliminate fear of specific situations before dismissal. He should display or verbalize the ability to analyze difficult situations and confirm the reduction of fear by frequent re-entries into these formerly dreaded situations.

### Postterminal Activities

The therapist has an obligation to follow up on his stutterers after they have been dismissed. It is not just a question of responsibility to certain individuals in the terminal stages of therapy; there are benefits to be gained in the form of increased knowledge of the effects of therapy. The more we know about the progress of our stutterers after therapy, the better able we are to predict the effect of therapeutic procedures on future clients. Too often we wave good-bye, wonder how the future will be, and then never see the child again. Responsible therapy demands adequate follow-up.

### Conferences

Postterminal activities are most frequently carried out through conferences with parents, teachers, and with the stutterers themselves. It is usually best to make definite appointments for future conferences at the final therapy session. During these conferences, the progress of the child's speech is checked directly or indirectly by questioning the parents and teachers. The parent is given the opportunity to present new problems that have arisen in seeking to provide an environment conducive to fluent speech. The therapist also has an opportunity to reinforce attitudes and objectives when he feels the need.

### Checking Classroom Performance

Wherever possible, observations of the child in situations outside of the clinic should be arranged. One of the best and frequently most convenient situations in which to observe the child is in his classroom. The therapist should arrange to be in the classroom at times when the child will be talking and, if possible, to be in an unobtrusive location. Plans should be made with the child's teacher to call on the child for oral recitation during the visit.

### Clarifying Roles

It is important that the part to be played by the teachers and parents during the postterminal stage is made clear to them. In addition to ascertaining their understanding of the factors involved in maintaining a climate suitable for continued fluent speech, the therapist should clarify their responsibilities in such activities as checking the child's speech or reminding him of things to be done. If the disfluencies are to be completely ignored, this should be made clear. On the other hand, if the child is to be reminded to enter particular speech situations, such should be known by the adults responsible for the child.

### The Relapse

Despite the best intentions of the therapist, parent, teacher, and child, the stutterer who once appeared to be free from stuttering symptoms may revert to his old behaviors. Relapses appear to be much more common among the Phase Three and Phase Four stutterers than among children whose stuttering has not advanced so far. With careful handling, the child whose problem has reoccurred can be helped to benefit from what he learns from the relapse and can emerge stronger than before. Potentially, however, the return of stuttering behaviors is dangerous, in that, if not handled properly, the child may develop a resistance to future therapy. Special attention needs to be given to children who experience a return of the stuttering problem after therapy.

## Why It Happens

One of the most common reasons for the relapse, particularly in the older and more advanced stutterer, is the change in rewards that occurs once contact with the therapist is discontinued. The child returns to a world that says in effect, "Don't stutter—or if you do, hide it!" The child no longer has the benefit of the therapist's reassurance in meeting such challenges and in facing difficult situations. The immediate rewards experienced in getting through a tough situation by the use of some avoidance device leads to the increased use of avoidances and before long the child feels the same amount of dread in speaking as he did before therapy.

> This sixteen-year-old boy had been dismissed from therapy just three months earlier. He was beginning to stutter severely again. After a conference involving both the boy and his mother, the stutterer was seen alone. The first thing he said as soon as his mother left was, "Can you tell my mother again that it is all right for me to stutter so long as I work on it? I was doing pretty well when I was up here with you this summer, but as soon as I got home, she began pointing out all of my blocks and asking me if I hadn't learned anything at the speech clinic. I've begun to dread stuttering almost as much as I did before I came up here!"

Stuttering sometimes returns due to overexpectations of fluency on the part of the child or his parents. Their basic fear of abnormal behavior and the relief experienced once speech has become more fluent leads them to develop unrealistic expectations of future fluency. Instead of noticing how much better the child is than when first brought to the clinic, many parents and stutterers begin looking for complete fluency, a phenomenon absent in the speech of even the most perfect orator. Such perfectionism can easily result in abnormal demands for fluency and tense reactions to the occurrence of disfluencies.

Some return of stuttering is not, in reality, a relapse, even though others may consider it as such. Natural variations in fluency occur even among speakers never labelled as stutterers.

Often normal disfluencies are seized upon and thought to be an indication that the effects of therapy are no longer operative. In such cases, reassurance and counseling usually suffice.

## Failure Trauma

Particularly among older stutterers, the first return of stuttering after therapy sometimes causes panic. Confidence gained slowly and gradually during therapy is shaken in a sudden and serious way. One stutterer whose progress had been steady and certain reached just such a panic stage while presiding at a club meeting shortly after therapy. The occurrence of one difficult word led to the sudden fear that her stuttering was returning. This fear gripped her so strongly that she had difficulty completing the meeting. Stuttering led to more stuttering and eventually to a tearful, disfluent phone call to her therapist requesting emergency help.

Failure trauma may be less dramatic but potentially more dangerous when it results in dejection and a feeling of hopelessness. This is especially likely to happen when an individual has so gradually slipped back into the use of avoidances that they resume full strength before he is even conscious of using them. Stuttering and the handicap of being different are then thought to be permanent and irreversible characteristics. Even if therapy is attempted in the future, the past reoccurrence of stuttering unconsciously reminds the individual that he cannot really expect to succeed. Some of the most difficult therapy problems arise out of a history of therapy success followed by relapse. The "defeatist attitude" really reaches its depth when "failure" follows "success."

## How to Handle the Relapse

The therapist has a responsibility to the stutterer, to future therapists, and to himself to attempt a successful solution to the problem of the child whose stuttering behavior has returned. One of the strongest emotional factors related to relapse is the feeling of guilt. The child feels guilty because he feels he has disappointed his parents and his therapist. The older stutterer has been told that stuttering is something he does and has control over so the return of stuttering signifies to him that he is not doing what he should—and yet he feels incapable of doing otherwise. The parents of the young stutterer have their problems too. These parents have

learned that stuttering is due, at least in part, to tensions created
in the home. A reoccurrence of disfluent speech is to them a sign
they are "bad parents." The therapist often shares some of this
guilt feeling because he thinks that if he had been wiser he might
have delayed the ending of therapy.

One of the first tasks of the therapist is to relieve these strong
feelings and establish a realistic approach which substitutes responsibility and thoughtful action for guilt and defensiveness. It
usually helps to encourage the individuals to air their grievances.
Sometimes this ventilation may be accelerated by bringing up
the subject directly and pointing out that these feelings are
normal and to be expected. Sometimes, a posture of calm waiting
and listening is enough to safely discharge these pent-up emotions.
Verbal attacks on the therapist should be recognized for what
they are—an attempt by the parent or child to avoid blame. It is
equally important for the therapist to be careful that his own guilt
does not lead to blame-avoidance tactics such as uttering the "If you
had only tried harder" type of statement.

Ventilation should be accompanied by reassurance. Recognition
is made again of the complexity of stuttering. No one has all the
answers. The most we can do is to reanalyze and start again with
the problem as it now stands.

Parents and children both need to realize that a return of disfluency does not necessarily mean a return of the total severity of
the problem. Many of the attitudes that will lead to eventual reduction of the problem may still be possessed and can still operate
to decrease the overt stuttering. A relapse does not mean that what
has been learned has been completely lost. Perhaps only reinforcement is necessary.

A careful reappraisal of the present status of the child's speech
should be made. Analysis of the overt stuttering behaviors may
reveal particular symptoms which require eradication. A survey
of the child's difficult situations may lead to the discovery of communicative pressures which have returned or which were never
modified. The evaluation of attitudes possessed by the child or
his parents and teachers may indicate the necessity for further conferences and discussion sessions. The therapist's task is to evaluate
the total problem and initiate a program designed to meet the
needs of the situation as it presently stands—not as it is hoped it
might be.

### Termination of "Unsuccessful" Cases

It is sometimes necessary to terminate therapy before the child's speech is considered rehabilitated. As is the case when apparently successful therapy is followed by a subsequent return of stuttering behaviors, the therapist has certain obligations to fulfill.

#### Clarification of Dismissal

All of the persons involved in a child's therapy should understand the basis of the decision to terminate and, in fact, should help make the decision if possible. It should be emphasized that the child's lack of progress is not a deliberate refusal on his part to cooperate with the therapy plan. Perhaps it is a sign that he cannot tolerate the experience of therapy at this time. The necessity of facing his stuttering at regular therapy sessions sometimes creates more anxiety than is dissipated during the therapy session. Some persons find it difficult to change, especially when there are rewards involved in continuing a behavior even though it also has its negative aspects. Some people are caught up in situations which defy modification and in which a high degree of tension is perpetuated in all areas of life. Stuttering sometimes is the lesser of several evils in these instances and may be the best or only outlet for excess anxiety.

#### Referrals

The unsuccessful case often requires other kinds of help. The child may need to be referred to another speech therapist. Frequently, referral to a psychologist or psychiatrist is indicated. Referral should not be left to chance. If the need exists, the therapist should assume the responsibility for making definite, specific referrals and for providing the referral source with pertinent information about the necessity for the referral.

#### Provision for Re-enrollment

Where therapy is terminated due to insufficient progress, the door must be kept open for future re-entry. Whenever possible, the parents should be told some of the signs to look for that will indicate a more favorable time to return to systematic therapy. Regular and frequent re-examinations or conferences should be scheduled so that a convenient avenue is available for re-enrollment.

*Unrecognized Success*

No one likes to fail or to end on failure. Therapists who experience this may find comfort in the fact that many stutterers whose therapy was considered unsatisfactory turned out later to be more successful than originally predicted. Many return at later times ready and able to make definite improvement in their speech. One of the authors dismissed a teen-ager several years ago. He had been in therapy for a long time and had apparently attained as much fluency as was possible at the time, even though he still experienced frequent, tense, stuttering blocks. The therapist moved to another state and lost contact with the boy. Recently, the stutterer —now a married adult—came to see the author to tell this story.

> You know, speech therapy really changed my life. I've been able ever since to do the things I was afraid of. My speech has gradually improved to the point where I seldom think of stuttering. Last year, though, my little girl began to stutter and was I scared! But I remembered what you had told me about normal stutterings and how calling attention to them made them worse so we just slowed down and tried to ignore them. She's doing all right now and so am I.

### References

1. AINSWORTH, S. *Speech Correction Methods* (Englewood Cliffs, N.J.: Prentice-Hall, Inc., 1948).
2. KENT, L. R. "A Retraining Program for the Adult Who Stutters," *Journal of Speech and Hearing Disorders,* XXVI (1961), 141-44.
3. *On Stuttering and Its Treatment* (Memphis, Tenn.: Speech Foundation of America, 1960).
4. SIEGENTHALER, B. M., and M. G. FLAMM. "Subjects' Self-Judgments of Speech Adequacy and Judgments by Trained Observers," *Journal of Speech and Hearing Disorders,* XXVI (1961), 244-51.
5. ———, A. J. DAVIS, and N. J. CHRISTENSEN. "Speech Ratings and Dismissal from Therapy," *Journal of Speech and Hearing Disorders,* XXVII (1962), 47-53.

# Chapter Eight

## Stuttering Modification in a
## Public School Setting

*This chapter is of concern to the speech therapist who is or will be engaged in speech therapy in a public school setting. The main emphasis is on a working relationship between the speech therapist and other school personnel and especially the transmission of pertinent information about stuttering and its modifications to the teacher directly responsible for the instruction of a young child who stutters.*

### Cooperation Between the Teacher and Speech Therapist

One of the authors had as a student in one of his classes a sixty-five-year-old woman, who, almost fifty years before, had taught for several years without a college degree and had been called back into active teaching during the critical shortage of teachers after World War II. She was taking one last course to complete her baccalaureate requirements. The day after graduation she planned to retire from teaching. During one of several enjoyable conversations with her, she brought out the following:

> Since returning to college, I have heard a great deal about the proper way of handling children who have problems. Most of my instructors claim that these approaches are based on research. Well, when I started teaching, we didn't approach the children statistically —*when they were troubled we simply put an arm around them. As I recall, we got good results.*

The wisdom of her remarks should not be overlooked. Basic to any healthy teacher-child relationship is mutual respect; a warm friendly teacher who earnestly tries to understand a child's problems serves as a source of strength immeasurably helpful to any child. As professional people, teachers are extremely conscious of their responsibilities to the children assigned to their care. Because of their direct responsibilities to children who stutter they often seek the aid of the school speech therapist because of the obvious need for a cooperative effort aimed at the welfare of a given child. The good therapist does the same, that is, seeks the aid of the child's teacher, but, in order that the child benefit fully, cooperation must be complete.

Perhaps the most important thing that needs to be said about the working relationship between the speech therapist and the classroom teacher is simply that they need each other. Working together they can cut down on the margin of error in their judgment about what is the best approach for a given child. A speech therapist can profit from the experience the classroom teacher has garnered from daily contact with normal children who have

their own share of non-speech-centered problems. The classroom
teacher is in the best possible position to observe daily changes
in the child's behavior. She will know what goes on on the play-
ground and in the cafeteria—who the child admires—and who he
is intimidated by. The clinician can provide specialized types of
information, but both kinds of information need to be pooled
to guard against an unwise course of action.*

The speech therapist should assume the responsibility for establishing this working relationship. How well the therapist will
succeed and be accepted will depend, in large part, on the personality of the therapist. An attitude of "holier than thou" or
"I'm the specialist" obviously is an approach to avoid (3).

Edney suggests this approach for helping the clinician to encourage the classroom teacher to become a cooperating member
of the team:

> First, he will build what might be called "personal" relationships,
> the liking of one individual for another. Second, the speech cor-
> rectionist will build the kind of relationships that come from under-
> standing and appreciating what the others are trying to do. In
> line with this he helps the classroom teacher understand the work of
> speech correction (a) by asking for a few minutes in each of a
> series of teachers' meetings to explain the nature of handicaps and
> the techniques used in their correction, (b) by setting up a series
> of short lecture-discussion periods to which all teachers are invited,
> (c) by extending to the teacher an invitation to visit speech cor-
> rection class (even though it is necessary to adapt his schedule in
> order to reach certain persons), or (d) by conducting workshops for
> classroom teachers where there is a desire and a request for them.
> Also, the speech correctionist will want to know as much as possible
> about the classroom teacher's work. Therefore, he will request per-
> mission to visit classes, and also will eagerly seek information about
> classroom activities. Third, the speech correctionist will build the
> sort of relationship that results from observation of results. If the
> classroom teacher observes a striking improvement in even one child,
> she develops respect for the program. Reports of progress sent to the
> classroom teacher help also. Fourth, the speech correctionist will
> build the kind of relationship that comes from a clear understanding
> of mutual obligations. He will confer with the classroom teacher
> frequently in order to clarify what each can do in order to correct
> and improve the speech of the child (2:425-26).

---

* An elaboration of the vital necessity for cooperative planning and sharing
of responsibility can be found in an article by Wilbur A. Yauch, "Role of the
Speech Correctionist in the Public School," *Exceptional Children,* XVIII (1952),
97-101.

One reason for establishing a close-knit relationship with all teachers is that they can and often do serve as prime referral sources of children to the school therapy program. Even if a thorough screening program initiated the speech correction program in a given school or school district, new children often arrive during the school year from another school district or from out of state. Usually there is some delay in transferring the child's school records and unless the school authorities are notified by a child's parents before school entrance, the child's new classroom teacher may very well be the first one in the school system who is aware of a child's hesitancy or stutter. An especially close relationship should be established with kindergarten and first-grade teachers—especially a relationship which will permit a free exchange of information about children newly enrolled each year.

Problems sometimes arise in these relationships because a particular teacher feels that she can make an adequate diagnosis of stuttering or nonstuttering and can determine the best course for the child without seeking professional guidance. Some are supremely confident that their guidance will assure that a hesitant child will, in the atmosphere of their classrooms, find the security to overcome what shyness or awkwardness he may bring with him from home—and eventually arrive at fluency. Some are prone to find any indication of disfluency a sure sign of incipient stuttering.

Regardless of the strength of the teacher's conviction that she knows what to do, the speech therapist cannot abrogate his right to decide whether a child is stuttering enough to warrant special attention. The therapist should make it clear that during the first stages of stuttering it is not wise to arrive at a hasty decision about whether disfluencies are true signs of stuttering. Observable breakdowns in speech may indeed disappear as the strangeness of the classroom wears off or the child becomes accustomed to classroom routine. It may be necessary to arrange to keep the child under unobtrusive observation for the time being in his classroom. On the other hand, the clinician should accept full responsibility for the placement of a child in a special class if in the clinician's opinion the special class is necessary. But if the child is doing well in school, the therapist should not feel that he must enroll a child for speech therapy unless there is a clear-cut need for such service. The decision to subject a child to speech therapy sessions should not be undertaken lightly—the consequences are too great as the following illustrates:

> The new year . . . started off for me with the following letter from a good friend who is a speech correction supervisor. There seems no point in merely filing it away out of sight. I'd like to share it with as many others as possible: "A couple of weeks before Christmas a teacher related to me the following sad tale: In our school we have a speech correctionist who comes once a week, takes the children out to a special class for 30 minutes. I did not send a little girl, 6½ years of age, from my first grade, because she has spoken perfectly all year and *does not have a speech defect.* But her mother called the principal about her and the speech therapist came to my room to get her. 'Why?' I asked. 'Because she stutters,' the speech teacher replied. 'But she has *never* stuttered yet in school!'
>
> "The speech teacher insisted it would please the mother to have her child getting the advantages of the speech correction program, so I sent the child to the speech clinic. When she returned we heard her falter and hesitate for the first time in her classroom. The following week I sent her again. Upon her return we were having a 'sharing' period about Thanksgiving experiences. The little girl got up as usual, began with a smile, then blocked completely on the word 'turkey.' She struggled for quite a while, then she broke into tears and sobbed to her classmates, 'I can't say it because I *stutter!'*
>
> "You will fully realize how I feel about such a crime being commited under the name of speech correction. The pity is that thousands of kids across the country are being sent to such special group classes, the mere attendance, even if the word stutter is never used there, being sufficient to create most unfortunate disturbances. I related this incident at a meeting last week, and one teacher asked me how else it could have been treated!
>
> "Of course the problem in this case is, as usual, that average daily attendance in the corrective speech classes is the basis for financial reimbursement to the local district by the state. Had the speech therapist visited the home and treated the causes there where the stuttering appeared she could not have counted her time for excess cost reimbursement. She can count her time only if she spends it with the child, not if she spends it with the parents. Where are we going to wedge in with some revolutionary and drastic revisions of such static concepts of speech therapy?" (4:175)

## Helping the Teacher

One reaction that most classroom teachers have when one of their students stutters is concern over the possibility that something will be done that will inadvertently jeopardize the child's welfare. Such a child can even be a threat to a classroom teacher because she may feel that she is inadequately prepared to provide the special care such a problem entails. It is imperative that the speech therapist educate teachers thoroughly. This is a part of therapy. If neglected it may continue to create problems and even irreversible damage.

### The Teacher's Attitude

Whether the child's stuttering is incipient or full-fledged, the teacher's attitude toward the observable behavior is of vital importance. Teachers' attitudes vary, but if a given teacher has not observed much stuttering, is in awe of it, feels incapable of being objective about it, or finds it difficult to look at, it may be that specific kinds of information about stuttering and its management will permit more adequate reactions on her part.

The therapist should observe the teacher in her daily classroom work to see if she can deal adequately with the child's stuttering. If she can't, she should be tactfully encouraged to maintain an unflurried, calm, interested attitude when face to face with the child's outward symptoms of stuttering. She perhaps realizes that the other children in her room are prone to ape her behavior. If she is impatient, the other children will feel it is justifiable to be brusque or hurry the stuttering child. If she is embarrassed, they will find it in themselves to show pity or even contempt. This means that she should be encouraged to force herself to listen with an interested expression on her face to what the youngster is saying and above all to look at him. The speech therapist should keep in mind that his experiences as a speech clinician have perhaps caused him to forget that this is not an easy thing to do at first for a person who has not been around much stuttering. The therapist must therefore be patient and respect the classroom teacher's awe or uneasiness.

The classroom teacher may inquire if it will embarrass a child if she looks directly at his contortions. The teacher might be reminded that we all like people to look at us when we talk. We don't want them to stare blindly through us, of course. No one ever looks directly at the same spot on the speaker's face for a long period of time. We look at the speaker *naturally*. This is much

different from either the quick withdrawal of eye contact whenever the speaker stutters or the vacant stare of one who is trying too hard to maintain eye contact when he finds it difficult to listen to what is being said. She should be assured that the child's self-respect will go begging if she only nervously glances at him from time to time. It should be pointed out that it is not necessary to look a person squarely in the eye to give the appearance of looking at him. At a distance of ten to fifteen feet or more, just looking at any part of a person's face will give the appearance of eye-to-eye contact. A blind person is taught to turn his face in the direction of his speaker or audience. The sighted person is often caught off-guard because the blind person seems to be seeing. The stutterer is seldom sure of being able to hold his audience's attention once he starts to talk. If his audience is unwilling to give him undivided attention, he may find it more and more difficult to labor through his speaking efforts. This experiment in anti-eye-contact might be suggested: while talking to an adult normal speaker, maintain eye contact (or face contact) for a short time then deliberately break off and look over his or her shoulder while the speaker continues to talk. Invariably even the most loquacious speakers are bound to break off conversation to locate the interrupter.

Attitudes are not expressed through eye contact alone. Equanimity is derived in part from hope. To know that the prognosis can be good—that the child's behavior will not inevitably worsen—can help objectivity. The following kinds of information should be conveyed to the teacher, just as they would be to the child's parents:

1. According to present evidence, stuttering appears to be more a matter of excess tension and "lack of confidence" in speaking than of something wrong with the speech apparatus.
2. Anything the teacher can do to help the child feel generally more confident will probably help indirectly to reduce the stuttering problem.
3. Most children will vary considerably in how much they stutter. In general, they tend to stutter less in those situations in which they feel confident and accepted.
4. Sudden increases in stuttering, as may occur sometimes in a classroom, may be the result of many different factors and not necessarily a sign that the teacher is handling the problem incorrectly.
5. Stuttering does not appear to be related to intelligence. Furthermore, even though it is related to emotional factors, it reflects only imper-

fectly the child's home environment, his emotional stability, or his concern about the speech problem.

6. Children who stutter usually have the same desire to enter into class discussions as other children in the room. Some children, because of their insecurity about talking, may give the appearance of not wanting to engage in general classroom activities. The teacher may help by finding the types of speaking these children enjoy and arranging for them to talk more in such situations.

7. Situations demanding quick, specific responses are likely to be harder for the child than situations in which he can choose his own time for making comments.

Sometimes the teacher will be concerned that she is part of the problem rather than part of the solution. She may feel that lack of improvement is partly her fault. The therapist will be concerned about this because the teacher's concern may be transmitted to the child. She should be assured that the most that can be expected of her is that the child's speech does not get worse while he is in her room. Maintaining the status quo is a reasonable goal and sometimes even a difficult goal to maintain.

But what if a child's speech suddenly flares up and boils over in a veritable fit of contortions and splutterings? Adult stutterers when questioned about their in-school experiences frequently report that they don't recall stuttering very much for several years until things came to a head. Then they have vivid memories of very severe stuttering in a certain grade (the grade level varies from report to report). Some reports indicate mismanagement or a lack of understanding on the part of a given teacher, but, quite often, not much is said about a teacher being at the bottom of the trouble. This much can be said to and about individual teachers. A teacher may not have had much to do with the flare-up—or if she did it might have been that the child decided that she was the kind of person to protest to because he could draw from this teacher's strength, or stability, or understanding. The teacher needs help in understanding that as a child stumbles and bumbles along in his speech—sometimes for years—his tolerance of his stuttering may begin to shift as his frustrations grow. His awareness of his speech awkwardness and remembered embarrassment is cumulative whereas the concern about his stuttering manifested by others may ebb and flow within predictable limits. During his first years of stuttering there may have been plenty of signs of awareness of his stutterings from his various listeners and not just from his parents. As he grew

older, members of his audience, feeling perhaps that he may not be going to outgrow his problem after all, tended, out of politeness if nothing else, to conceal their concern about his stutterings. Over a period of years he may become more and more aware of the fact that *most people don't seem to pay much attention to the fact that he stutters.* Over a period of years the young stutterer also becomes increasingly aware that no matter how he twists and turns trying to detach himself from the shadow of his stuttering he more and more realizes that he cannot escape from it. His frustrations may come to a head because pressures finally become unbearable. The final straw is placed on his shoulders. He may have been led to believe that he would outgrow his problem. Indeed, both he and his parents have believed in this oft-told tale. Finally, he may find it necessary to dramatize his plight. The sudden increase in stutterings may be his way of signalling that he needs help or assurance. He may be signalling to his teacher (he will need someone to signal to) that if you haven't been noticing the way I struggle when I talk—then you should.

## How Much Talking?

The clinician should help the classroom teacher know that a child who stutters must have ample opportunity to talk. His teacher must realize that he should be encouraged to talk because skill and confidence in talking is acquired through continual practice. Also, even though he may be embarrassed by his stuttering when he talks, fear will grow more rapidly during his avoidance of talking. Fortunately the very young stutterer may not be in the least reluctant to talk, but as the burden of stuttering grows, there is a tendency for the amount of talking to decrease due to the cumulative effects of embarrassment or anxiety about possible embarrassment. Some children go so far as to completely refuse to talk. Sometimes routine classroom procedures prove to be too difficult for a stuttering child to cope with—especially those that necessitate adequate performance via talking.

## Oral Recitation

Johnson, in discussing classroom oral recitation problems, points out that a stutterer is vulnerable because stuttering is essentially an anxiety or fear response which tends to mount under conditions of suspense.

Fiction writers make the most of this fact, of course. The well-worn stories about expectant fathers illustrate the point elaborately. Now, one of the reasons why reciting in certain classrooms is so distressing to many stutterers is simply that it proceeds alphabetically, and the farther down the list from "A" the stutterer's name comes, the longer he has to worry about whether or not he will be able to answer—and the longer he worries, the greater his doubts and fears become and the more likely he is to stutter when his name is finally called. Pity the stuttering child whose name begins with "Z"! (5:44)

Knudson (8), in a study of the oral recitation problems of stutterers, found that sixty-two of the seventy-two stutterers interviewed felt that they made poorer oral recitations than their intellectual ability would warrant. Approximately 50 per cent admitted having said, "I don't know," or had given the wrong answer to avoid a feared word. Knudson points out that teachers should be especially cautious about reprimanding a student who refuses to recite or who gives the impression of being continually unprepared until the cause of the reticence is determined. In no instance is there justification for forcing a child to talk. Pushing a child into a forbidding speech situation is like pushing a nonswimmer who is afraid of water in over his head—the consequences are serious. But the nonswimmer can be taught to enjoy swimming, and the stutterer can learn the joys of talking, both by intelligent planning on the part of the teacher or the therapist.

Knudson suggests the following possible approaches to the oral recitation problems of stutterers:

Some students may not be able to give entire book reports or make long oral recitations until they have had more help with their speech. In severe instances it may not be wise or practical for either the student or the class. All stutterers, however, can give "yes" or "no" responses or very brief replies in order not to feel ignored or excluded from the group. This method will also hold them to a preparation of the subject matter; for, if a student is never called upon to recite, he loses the motivation to study and his grades suffer accordingly.

It is usually desirable to demand extra written work of the student to the extent that he is excused from oral recitation. Such a procedure is conducive to a more thorough preparation and a greater interest in his school work.

One plan that a number of stutterers seemed to favor was to call on them to recite only when they volunteered to do so. This plan, however, would need to be definitely agreed upon by both the teacher and the pupil. The stutterer would thus be relieved of the anxiety and mental strain of wondering when he would be called upon and he could give more attention to the subject matter at hand (7:46).

West, Ansberry, and Carr suggest that the best way to answer the question about whether the stutterer should be forced, encouraged, allowed, discouraged, or forbidden to recite orally is to repeat the statements of adult stutterers regarding the matter.

> An occasional adult stutterer will say that he liked a certain teacher because she never called on him. The majority, however, remember the acute embarrassment caused when the teacher never called upon them to recite or read aloud when all the other children were called upon regularly. One stutterer said: "One teacher thought she was being very clever. She always arranged it so that the paragraph I had to read was the shortest one on the page. She always called on me when we had what she thought was easy reading, or perhaps she would have me do an errand to the office during oral reading time. I hated that teacher. She made me feel like a fool! One of my teachers could never see my hand when I raised it after she had asked a question. Finally, I got so I either didn't study and raised my hand anyway, or I just quit raising it (10:434)."

## Helping with Words

Classroom teachers often ask if it will help a child to talk more if he is given help with his troublesome words. It should be pointed out that in almost every instance the child should be permitted to attempt and finish his own words without assistance.

However, there are some indirect ways of helping a child through a troublesome period. This is the way one speech therapist handled this particular kind of situation.

> One day while talking to a teacher about a child in her room who was stuttering, he recalls that he was quite shaken up when the teacher said that whenever the child had a particularly severe block she interrupted him and made him wait until he had calmed down before she let him go on talking. The speech therapist, formerly a severe stutterer himself, was relieved that he questioned her about her manner of interruption before he indicated his disapproval of interrupting a child in the middle of a block. She said that quite often the child would come up to her to ask her questions about assignments while she was standing by her desk. She said that if he started off pretty badly and that if she felt it was going to be a great

struggle for him to get the next word out she would casually put her arm around the child and say, "Wait just a moment please." Then looking out over his shoulder she would say to one of the other children, "John, would you open the window a little more," or "Several of you aren't working on your lesson."

Some children are adept at getting someone else to say their feared words. If this happens the speech therapist must point out that if the teacher allows this to continue she may be instrumental in helping him reinforce a pattern of habitual avoidance of words. Sometimes she may think she is helpfully supplying a word, whereas she may not be able to predict what he is trying to say too well and thus is only interrupting. Neely, in an interesting discussion of the stutterer's frustration prompted by the interrupting answer to his unfinished question, states: "A common entry in the list of complaints of people who stutter is the anticipating answer or the anticipated question. We who stutter dislike the teacher, girl friend, or teammate who engaged in this mind reading. We have aired our views often enough that a rule of thumb in clinical practice is: *Don't interrupt the stutterer* (9:165)."

He goes on to point out that because of the redundancy in our language (the *u*'s always following *q*'s in writing and the contextual redundancies in speaking, "Where are you g . . . ?) the normal speaker is also interrupted because we speak a redundant language. He suggests that although it is considered more polite to wait for the person to finish talking before we answer, those who stutter can learn to accept the interruptions more readily and in the spirit in which they are given if the redundant language of our society is made clear to them. But this approach may be one that the therapist would want to employ in direct therapy rather than suggesting it to the child's teacher.

### Teasing and Mocking

There may come a time when the teacher mentions that she has noticed a child being teased about his stuttering and wants suggestions about handling the situation. One way a teacher may offset this is to talk to the child or children doing the teasing or mocking. A conference can be arranged with the offender (the child who stutters should not be present) and in a friendly way it should be explained that the stuttering will change and even disappear if given a chance. It should be explained to the teaser that if the teasing is continued the stuttering may even become worse because of the teasing. The teacher can enlist the taunter's aid in seeing to it that other children refrain from making unkind remarks. If this plea is made patiently and calmly, but forcibly, the offending children will usually be reasonable about the matter.

An adult female stutterer whom we worked with reported that she had absolutely no recollection of ever having been teased about her stuttering by a classmate even though she had stuttered quite severely in school. One day Betty reported the following episode which points up a rather drastic approach to the prevention of teasing.

> Yesterday while downtown shopping I ran into a schoolmate whom I hadn't seen in years. This gave me an excellent chance to talk about the fact that I was attending the speech clinic and was working on my stuttering. She said she remembered my stuttering even early in grade school but she remembered most vividly the fact that Miss_____, who taught third grade, had talked to the whole class about it one day. Apparently I was out of the room because this is the first time I had any inkling of why nothing was ever said about my stuttering. Miss_____ apparently told the group that if anyone ever so much as looked crosseyed at me she would snatch them bald, and if you knew Miss_____, you'd know why it took me almost twenty-five years to find out. . . .

It will certainly help the child if he has some verbal way to defend himself against teasing or mockery. The child's teacher should be informed that the older child who looks upon himself as a stutterer can be taught constructive means of combating the overt rejection of his peers. It may be that in the therapy sessions the child has been encouraged to confront his tormentor with, "Sure I stutter—so what?" or "Yes, I stutter but one of these days I'll get over it." The teacher should know about this.

*The Stress on Fluency*

One of the problems facing a stutterer is the listener's rejection of disfluency. As has been pointed out before, even though a stutterer's speech may be intelligible—even though he expresses his ideas well—breaks in the rhythm of his speech patterns are often pounced upon as unforgivable lapses. The stutterer is often just as intolerant of these lapses as are his listeners. Dr. Wendell Johnson in *Stuttering and What You Can Do About It* (6) points out that it is important to listen for hesitations and repetitions in a child's speech that *should be regarded as normal* rather than to focus attention on disfluencies. He points out that this is a particularly effective aid in breaking up the vicious circle of hesitancy, concern, more hesitancy, more concern, etc.

Just as with the child's parents, the child's teacher should understand that under no circumstances is fluency at any price to be condoned. Especially deplorable is the suggestion of some very well-meaning people (and even some teachers) that if the young stutterer should employ some device or trick he will be able to talk more fluently. These devices or tricks usually consist of a nonspeech motor act timed with the disfluency so that a release will occur. They include: snapping or tapping fingers, licking lips, blinking eyes, taking a breath, tapping a toe, or others to initiate or terminate a troublesome word. Teachers should know that *these tricks or devices should never be taught to a child.* It should be pointed out that these mannerisms may help briefly, but in a short time their effectiveness wears off. The insidious thing about these tricks is that they do provide immediate relief. But, too often, when the tricks no longer help, they are not dropped but remain a habitual part of talking. Depending on the tricks he was taught, the child will eventually develop a bizarre pattern of blinking his eyes, snapping his fingers, or protruding his tongue when blocked—often the resulting behavior is more grotesque than if he had simply blundered his way through the word in the first place.

### Inform the Teacher of the Basic Rationale of Therapy

The speech therapist should make it clear to the teacher that as stuttering becomes more and more chronic, the stuttering tends to stem more and more from the stutterer's attempts to keep from stuttering. Successful speech therapy often results in more fluency and fewer and less severe moments of stuttering. But the child's teacher must be informed about the objectives of therapy—especially that speech therapy is not aimed at fluency alone. She must be aware that in the first stages of therapy fluency may appear spontaneously. This "false fluency" may be the direct result of the emphasis in therapy on "stuttering out in the open"—the antithesis of hiding or avoiding moments of stuttering. Teachers must be aware of the fact that in this stage of therapy a child's fears of stuttering are counteracted and materially reduced by encouraging the child to stutter and that when he is rewarded he is rewarded for stuttering without avoidance—his rewards do not stem from the therapist's approval of fluency.

The opposite reaction often occurs too. Due to the withdrawal of tricks and the increased emphasis upon the speech pattern, stuttering often increases in severity at the early stages of therapy. The child's teacher (and his parents) should be forewarned of this possibility so that their reaction is not too great. So long as they understand that the increased disfluency is a temporary condition, they will be able to accept it.

Teachers should know that in speech therapy no premium is placed on fluency (at least at first) because this may reinforce the drive that maintains the stuttering. The teacher should be helped to realize that if she praises a child for talking without stuttering she may emphasize the undesirability of his stuttering. As Bloodstein has pointed out, stuttering is a child's conscientious effort to speak acceptably despite a deep conviction that he cannot do so (1:38). This deep conviction that he cannot speak acceptably may be due to the fact that he ardently wishes to please his parents and his teachers with the only type of speech they seem to want— fluent speech. The teacher must be helped to know that if she wishes the therapy program to be successful she simply must not emphasize the all-importance of fluency.

## How to Praise the Stuttering Child

Once the child achieves some measure of fluency he is too often confronted with praise expressed in these words: *I certainly am pleased with the way you are talking. I knew you could talk this way. Now if you keep on trying the way you are, I know you'll be able to lick this.*

If the teacher expresses her approval in this way, it will help to point out to her that these kinds of remarks do several things to a child—all of them undesirable. First they point up again that the appraiser objects to stuttering. Secondly, "I knew you could," suggests that the person doing the appraising knows a great deal about the stutterer and implies that he knows a lot more things that he could do—if he only would. Thirdly, they contain an implied threat, "Be sure you keep on trying to talk this way if you want my continued approval." The appraiser doesn't necessarily mean to have his remarks interpreted in this way but far too often this is the way they get interpreted because they are directed at a person who (a) doesn't like to stutter, (b) wishes he knew enough about himself to break through his disfluency barrier, and (c) wants to keep in the good graces of his listeners.

The speech therapist must draw on as many resources as possible to help the beholder of the stuttering realize the futility of denouncing the block. The clinician should explain that it is far more rewarding and profitable if praise can be directed at a stutterer's attempt to let the block come out without struggle or avoidance. It is much more rewarding to the stuttering child if his listener will remain objective about his disfluencies. Listener eye contact and patience are often more helpful than are comments concerning fluency.

An extension of "I knew you could," is "I suppose you realize that I know of many other things you can do." It is utterly futile to attempt to maintain the approval of this kind of person because he hasn't indicated acceptance—he has only indicated that the stutterer has taken the first step of an indefinite number of steps that may *eventually* lead to approval. A more suitable phrase—one that would indicate awareness of growth, change, or an attempt at new behavior—is "Well, I'll be darned!" In effect this says, "Do you mean to tell me that *you* did that? I guess there is nothing for me to do but change my opinion of you." This kind of statement says in effect, "What you are doing is pretty hard to do and although I didn't really expect it of you, I learn new things about you every day."

### Perspective

Much of the content of this chapter is a digest of what has already been discussed in this book. But the teacher must have this information. Not only the teacher, but also parents, principals, superintendents, and physicians need such knowledge. It is imperative that these things be said. How it is said is important also. It shouldn't be told all at once, nor should the teacher be hammered with it so hard that she becomes thoroughly impressed with her potential for doing wrong. If told too well too strongly, the teacher may not be able to be at ease and relaxed in the face of a child's stuttering. The information can be conveyed piecemeal. Sometimes brief exchanges with the teacher at the classroom door when returning a child to his room after a therapy session will do the job. Regularly scheduled conferences with teachers who have stuttering children permit a more systematic presentation. This information is important enough to serve as a topic for a series of in-service meetings for all teachers and school nurses.* Parent groups, PTA, women's clubs, and service organizations need to know about stuttering and what can be done to prevent it and what can be done for it once it is a reality.

As mentioned in previous chapters, there is a difference in how receptive different individuals are to our counseling. Some of this receptivity—either positive or negative—is uncontrollable from the therapist's standpoint. Receptivity, however, is due directly to the manner in which the therapist handles his public relations. Keeping in mind that the child who stutters is the key figure in the problem, the therapist needs to strive continually to secure the best possible interrelationships with teachers, principals, and others. The therapist must frequently remind himself that the best chances for success with the child are found when all important adults are working together for the child's benefit.

### References

1. BLOODSTEIN, O. "Stuttering as an Anticipatory Struggle Reaction," in J. Eisenson (ed.), *Stuttering: A Symposium* (New York: Harper & Row, Publishers, 1958).
2. EDNEY, C. W. Chapter 9, "The Public School Remedial Speech Program," in *Speech Handicapped School Children,* Revised Ed. (New York: Harper & Row, Publishers, 1956).
3. IRWIN, R. B. *Speech and Hearing Therapy* (Englewood Cliffs, N.J.: Prentice-Hall, Inc., 1954).
4. JOHNSON, W. "Letters to the Editor," *Journal of Speech and Hearing Disorders,* XIV (1949), 175.
5. ————, et al. *Speech Handicapped School Children,* Revised Ed. (New York: Harper & Row, Publishers, 1956).
6. ————. *Stuttering and What You Can Do About It* (Minneapolis: University of Minnesota Press, 1961).
7. KNUDSON, T. A. "Stuttering," in the issue "Speech and Hearing Problems in the Secondary-School," *The Bulletin of the National Association of Secondary-School Principals,* XXXIV (1950), 40-48.

---

* For more information on how to conduct an in-service training program see Chapter 9, "In-Service Training," in Ruth B. Irwin's *Speech and Hearing Therapy* (Englewood Cliffs, N.J.: Prentice-Hall, Inc., 1954).

8. ———. "A Study of the Oral Recitation Problems of Stutterers," *Journal of Speech Disorders*, IV (1939), 235-39.
9. NEELY, K. "Letters to the Editor," *Journal of Speech and Hearing Disorders*, XVI (1951), 165-66.
10. WEST, R., M. ANSBERRY, and A. CARR. *The Rehabilitation of Speech*, Third Ed. (New York: Harper & Row, Publishers, 1957).

# Appendix A

## Stuttering: Diagnostic and
### Evaluative Checklist

Name _____ Sex ____ Birthdate _____ Age ____
Parents' Names _____
Parents' Address _____
School _____ Grade ____ Teacher _____
Phase:  1  2  3  4  (Circle one)

*Characteristics and Distinguishing Features of Problem:*

Etiologic Factors:

Psychometric Information:

Medical Information:

1. *Fluent Periods:*
   Chronic _____     Episodic _____
   Duration _____    Length of recent episodes of rela-
                                 tive fluency:
   _____             Day(s) _____
   _____             Week(s) _____
   _____             Month(s) _____

2. *Awareness or emotionality:*
   Symptoms referred to as:
   Parent _____
   Child _____
   Evidence of embarrassment or anxiety:
   Parent _____

   Child _____

   Eye Contact:   Good ( )   Fair ( )   Poor ( )

3. *Repetitions* (clonic):
   _____ Deliberate, effortless, unhurried
   _____ Hurried, rapid bursts
   Duration _____
   Words ( )   Syllables ( )   Sounds ( )
       Position in sentence: Initial ( )   Indeterminate ( )
       Word types:
       _____ Small connective or relational words
       _____ Major words

4. *Hard Contacts or Prolongations* (tonic):
_____ Tense—forceful attack
Tremor _____
_____ Easy—low pressure
Tension loci _____

Duration _____

Other _____

5. *Interjections of extraneous words, sounds, or phrases:*
_____ Before first word in sentence
_____ Between words in sentence
Nature of interjection _____

6. *Consistency and Adaptation:*
My name is _____ (child's name).
I like to run and jump.
Some trees lose their leaves in winter.
Birds fly very high in the sky.
We sometimes watch football in the afternoon.
We had a nice long ride in a sailboat.
We may get wet if it starts to rain.
Somebody told him to open the package when he got home.

7. *Associated Tension of Respiratory Mechanism:*
_____ Exaggerated pausing
_____ Speaking on residual air
_____ Violent gasping
_____ Others

8. *Movement of Extremities:*
_____ Clenching fists
_____ Hiding mouth with hand
_____ Striking mouth with hand
_____ Grasping the chin
_____ Kicking out with foot
_____ Others

9. *Facial Tension:*
_____ Eye blinking        _____ Opening mouth
_____ Eye closure         _____ Protrusion of the tongue
_____ Eye dilation        _____ Twisting of the mouth
_____ Eye rolling         _____ Flaring of nostrils
_____ Frowning            _____ Others
_____ Jaw jerk

10. *Tension of Torso:*
  _____ Bending body
  _____ Jerking body
  _____ Rigidity of body
  _____ Others

11. *Head Movement:*
  _____ Up—down—sideways
  _____ Other

12. *Prespasm Activities:*
  A. *Avoidance:*
    _____ Substitution of another word
    _____ Giving up speech attempt altogether
    _____ Changing the order of the words
    _____ Waiting for help on the word
    _____ Pretending to think
    _____ Evasion through rationalization, "I don't know," etc.
    _____ Communicating by gestures, writing, etc.
    _____ Others
  B. *Postponement:*
    _____ Use of ah, oh, or irrelevant words, to delay speech attempt
    _____ Sub-vocal rehearsal
    _____ Pausing, pretending to think
    _____ Circumlocution—talking around word to delay speech attempt
    _____ Repeating previous words or phrases
    _____ Others
  C. *Starters:*
    _____ Use of timing devices—eye blinks, head or jaw jerks, hand movements, etc.
    _____ Increasing rate of speech
    _____ Back up to get running start
    _____ Exhalation—residual air
    _____ Use of oh, ah, um, etc., to get word started
    _____ Use of stereotyped movement before speech attempt (body jerk, swallowing, eye blink, etc.)
    _____ Sudden increase of tension and force
    _____ Others
  D. *Anti-Expectancy:*
    _____ Using a kind of speech in which no word stands out enough to be feared, such as: monotone, slow deliberate, singing, rapid, or slurred speech
    _____ Filling the mind with other things so that the expectancy of stuttering is kept out (distraction)
    _____ Assuming an attitude of self-confidence; assumption of aggressive, belligerent, clowning behavior; whispered re-

hearsal; compensatory behavior of various kinds; use of coughing or some such obvious activity

_____ Others

13. *Release Mechanisms:*

_____ Finish block using some starter, timing, or other blockbusting device

_____ Cease speech attempt and try again

_____ Stop and use some distraction

_____ Stop and assume a change in attitude

_____ Others

14. *Postspasm Reaction:*

_____ Ignore block entirely

_____ Laugh, show indifference or bravado

_____ Display humiliation, embarrassment

_____ Desire to run away from situation

_____ Talk fast

_____ Others

*Appendix B*

## Special Case History (Stuttering)

This information can be obtained from the child's parents, guardians, or teachers, or other people important to the child. This particular form is designed to be filled out by the person from whom the information is being solicited in the informant's own writing. It is unwise, however, to try to obtain information in this way unless the person has directly expressed an interest in helping "in any way possible." This form can be used conveniently as a guide in a face-to-face interview.

Name of child _____

Name of person providing information _____

Relationship to child _____ Date _____

Please describe his way of talking in your own words:

_____

_____

_____

Do you have any idea how his stuttering started? _____

_____

When was his stuttering first noticed? By whom? _____

_____

Does he show signs of being concerned or embarrassed about his way of talking (crying, refusing to talk, claiming he can't say certain words, getting red in the face, stamping his foot, not answering the door or telephone, avoiding strangers, etc.)? _____

_____

_____

Was he late in learning to talk? Please describe. _____

_____

Have any of his relatives stuttered? If so, who? _____

What special means have been taken by you or anyone else to help him get over his stuttering? _____

Does he have trouble getting along with anyone in the family? If so please describe. _____

Has his speech improved or worsened lately? _____

What are his special interests ( hobbies, pets, favorite sports or activities, clubs, possessions, etc.)? _____

How concerned are you about his way of talking? _____

# Appendix C

## General Case History

(Confidential)

Please answer every question to the best of your knowledge. If possible, please return this form to the Center so that it may be reviewed before the first interview.

Name of Case _____ Birthdate _____ Age ____ Sex ____
Address of Case _____ Date of First Appointment _____
Address of Parent _____ Phone _____
   or Guardian

Do not write in this space

Nature

Etiology

Rapport

Prognosis

Recommendations

## Family History

| Name | Age | Speech Defect | Other Information |

Father _____

Mother _____

Brothers _____

Sisters _____

Other Relatives _____

Other Relatives Living at Home _____

Family Religion _____

Which parent does child prefer _____ Why _____

Which brother or sister does child prefer _____ Why _____

## Speech History

Description of speech problems in your own words _____

_____

_____

At what age did child say simple words _____ Phrases _____

Do you associate the speech difficulty with any severe illness or unusual
occurance _____

_____

What throat or mouth diseases or injuries has the child had _____

At what age was speech difficulty first noticed _____

Is the child hard of hearing _____

Has the child ever had more speech than he has now _____

Has the child's speech shown any improvement lately _____

Has the patient previously been examined or received therapy for speech
problem _____ Where _____

_____ When _____ By whom _____

_____ Recommendations or treatment given _____

_____

Remarks _____

_____

_____

### Developmental History

Type of feeding as infant ＿＿＿＿＿＿ Any problems ＿＿＿＿＿＿

Was the child's rate of growth seemingly normal ＿＿＿＿＿＿
If not, describe ＿＿＿＿＿＿＿＿＿＿＿＿＿＿

Give age at which following took place: First tooth ＿＿＿＿＿＿
Full set of teeth ＿＿＿＿＿＿ Full set of second teeth ＿＿＿＿
First sat alone ＿＿＿＿＿＿ Crawled ＿＿＿＿＿＿ Walked ＿＿＿＿
Fed self ＿＿＿＿＿＿ Dressed self ＿＿＿＿＿＿＿＿＿

Which hand does the child use Right ＿＿＿＿＿＿ Left ＿＿＿＿＿
Ambidextrous ＿＿＿＿＿＿＿＿＿＿＿＿＿

Has handedness ever been changed ＿＿＿＿ When ＿＿＿＿＿＿

Has the child ever written backwards ＿＿＿＿ When ＿＿＿＿＿＿

Childhood problems: Indicate how often these problems occur by encircling the letter which most clearly describes. "O" indicates "often," "S" indicates "seldom."

| | | | | | | |
|---|---|---|---|---|---|---|
| Nightmares | O S | Nervousness | O S | Walking in sleep | O S |
| Shyness | O S | Sleeplessness | O S | Refusal to eat | O S |
| Showing off | O S | Bed wetting | O S | Face twitching | O S |
| Strong fears | O S | Constipation | O S | Temper tantrums | O S |
| Whining | O S | Thumb sucking | O S | Destructiveness | O S |
| Strong hates | O S | Running away | O S | Smoking | O S |
| Rudeness | O S | Tongue sucking | O S | Selfishness | O S |
| Jealousy | O S | Hurting pets | O S | Stealing | O S |
| Lying | O S | Setting fires | O S | Fainting | O S |
| Playing with sex organs | . . . . . . . . . . . . O S | Queer food habits | O S |

### Birth History

Age of mother at time of birth ＿＿＿＿＿＿ Age of father ＿＿＿＿＿

Conditions during pregnancy (working, health, shocks or accidents, medical care, etc.) ＿＿＿＿＿＿＿＿＿＿＿＿＿
＿＿＿＿＿＿＿＿＿＿＿＿＿＿＿＿＿
＿＿＿＿＿＿＿＿＿＿＿＿＿＿＿＿＿

Was the delivery normal ＿＿＿＿＿＿ Prolonged ＿＿＿＿＿＿
Instruments used ＿＿＿＿＿＿ Caesarean ＿＿＿＿＿＿ Was there
evidence of injury at birth (describe) ＿＿＿＿＿＿＿＿＿
＿＿＿＿＿＿＿＿＿＿＿＿＿＿＿＿＿

### Physical Condition of Child

Height ＿＿＿＿＿＿ and weight ＿＿＿＿＿＿ of child at present time.
Any physical deformities ＿＿＿＿＿＿＿＿＿

Main findings of last physical examination ＿＿＿＿＿＿＿＿
＿＿＿＿＿＿＿＿＿＿＿＿＿＿＿＿＿

Dr. ＿＿＿＿＿＿ Address ＿＿＿＿＿＿ Date＿＿＿＿＿

Check diseases he has had, giving age and severity. "M" indicates mild, "A"—average, "S"—severe.

| *Diseases* | *Age* | | | | *Diseases* | *Age* | | | |
|---|---|---|---|---|---|---|---|---|---|
| Tonsilitis | | M | A | S | Pneumonia | | M | A | S |
| Whooping cough | | M | A | S | Pleurisy | | M | A | S |
| Scarlet fever | | M | A | S | Influenza | | M | A | S |
| Typhoid fever | | M | A | S | Diphtheria | | M | A | S |
| Tuberculosis | | M | A | S | Mumps | | M | A | S |
| Chicken pox | | M | A | S | Rickets | | M | A | S |
| German measles | | M | A | S | Rheumatism | | M | A | S |
| Measles | | M | A | S | Dysentery | | M | A | S |
| St. Vitus Dance | | | | | Bronchitis | | M | A | S |
| (chorea) | | M | A | S | Croup | | M | A | S |
| Convulsions | | M | A | S | Earache | | M | A | S |
| Enlarged glands | | M | A | S | High fever | | M | A | S |
| Heart trouble | | M | A | S | Encephalitis | | | | |
| Thyroid disturbances | | M | A | S | (brain fever) | | M | A | S |
| Infantile paralysis | | M | A | S | Convulsions—associated | | | | |
| Appendicitis | | M | A | S | with fever | | M | A | S |
| Frequent colds | | M | A | S | Convulsions—not associ- | | | | |
| | | | | | ated with fever | | M | A | S |
| | | | | | Any other | | M | A | S |

Remarks _____

Has the child ever been seriously injured or had a severe shock _____
State nature of injury or shock, age, and effects _____

Has the child had any operations (tonsils, adenoids, tongue tie, palate repair, etc.) _____

Approximate date _____ Surgeon _____

#### Educational History

Is the child average _____, below average _____, or
superior _____ in intelligence.
Are school marks average _____ below average _____
or above average _____
Has the child ever failed or skipped a grade in school _____
Present grade _____
Schools attended and dates (include nursery and kindergarten) _____
_____
_____

Does the child like school _____ If not, why _____
_____

## Social Development

Does the child have opportunity for regular play with children _____
  What ages _____ How many _____
Is the child usually follower or leader _____
Does child fight frequently with playmates _____
Does he prefer to play alone _____
Which playmates does the child prefer _____ Why _____

_____

_____

_____

# Index